VISION ASSESSMENT
of
Infants & Children
with & without
Special Needs

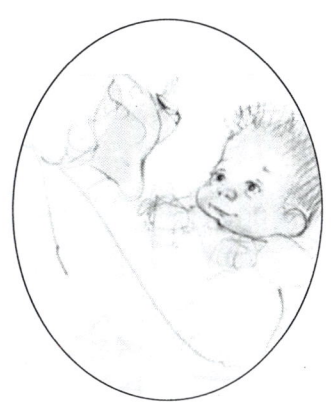

PART 1
Functional Vision Assessment of Infants & Special Needs Children

Useful for: Vision Teachers, Therapists, and University Training Programs...

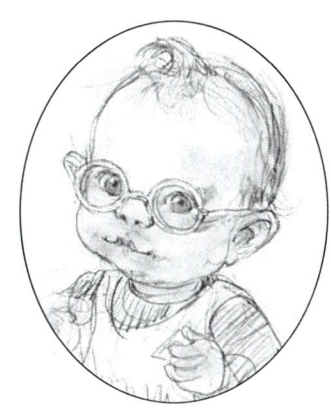

PART 2
Baby Vision Screening with Play

Useful for: Baby Programs Mandated to Screen Birth to 3 Year Olds

VISION ASSOCIATES
2109 W US HWY 90 STE 170-312
Lake City, FL 32055-7708

Introduction

Greetings ..... to all of you involved with assessing vision in infants and children with "special" needs, not an easy task, but one that is important and especially rewarding when visual information is uncovered. Remember you're not alone. We were all beginners at one time. The more children you assess the more skilled you will become and the more comfortable you will be with assessing vision.

Far too many children miss receiving necessary and thorough visual examinations. Identifying visual deficits utilizing a "team" approach can minimize this. The "team" may include ophthalmologists, optometrists, vision teachers, therapists, vision screeners, other medical professionals and parents/guardians. If after completion of functional vision assessments and/or vision screenings there are visual concerns, it is important to follow your programs procedure in referring the child to the appropriate doctor for a complete vision evaluation.

This book was written in two parts with the goals of sharing practical information and a reference for offering vision assessment and vision screening suggestions. It is not intended to be an in depth "training" guide. If this is your need I suggest you check out, "ISAVE-Individualized Systematic Assessment of Visual Efficiency" by M. Beth Langley (1998). This publication is amazingly detailed and filled with great, in depth, information.

If vision assessment and screening are new to you I suggest you use the references in the Appendix as part of your learning to gain information from the "movers and shakers" in the educational and medical vision world. In addition, it is advisable that you find an experienced vision assessment person to assist in your training.

PART 1 includes background information on assessment of infants and special needs children, an overview of the visual system, tips and procedure of assessment and recording and reporting forms. It was written for people who have some vision background, such as vision teachers and/or therapists.

Greetings also to those of you who are responsible for screening vision of babies based on the legislative mandates requiring all infants referred for early intervention services to receive timely and comprehensive multidisciplinary evaluations and assessments, including vision. I have often thought about how to assist you with this awesome task. I realize not all of you have a vision background, so I kept PART 2 simple and to the point including step by step guidelines, suggested toys or tests to use and recording and feedback forms. Hopefully you will find this helpful in accomplishing your goals.

As a vision teacher I am aware of how important it is to learn about children's functional vision and how eclectically assessment knowledge is obtained. My vision assessment background was gathered through education, training, assessing vision, tagging along with skilled peers, and working closely with ophthalmologists and optometrists. In addition, I have admired and learned from many excellent vision educational professionals over the years.

When I began doing vision assessments I was unclear as to <u>what to do</u> with the out comes of assessments and <u>how to</u> develop intervention goals based on assessment. Thanks to a variety of doctors I took new paths on the assessment journey and began learning about the visual system and how it relates to function. Vito Racanneli, OD, was the doctor who taught me "tricks of the trade" and suggested that often the best way to assess "special needs" children is lying on the floor. Lea Hyvärinen, MD led me in many directions including learning about contrast sensitivity and acuity testing, but her work and research pertaining to the brain and vision has been an extremely important path. Dr. Jim Jan's work and research has led us all to better understanding of Cortical Vision Impairment, and Mitchell Scheiman, OD smoothed out many bumps in the road toward better understanding of vision efficiency. You will find many references to their work in this book.

It is interesting to note that the American Academy of Ophthalmology recommends: <u>newborns</u> be examined by pediatricians or family physicians and examined by ophthalmologists, at appropriate intervals, if infants are at high risk. Infants at <u>6 months</u> of age should be screened for ocular health by pediatricians, family physicians or ophthalmologists. At about <u>3 1/2 years</u> of age children should be screened for eye health by pediatricians, family physicians, or ophthalmologists, emphasizing acuity. At age <u>5 years</u> children should have vision evaluations including alignment by pediatricians, family physicians or ophthalmologists. Further screenings should be done at school checks or if symptoms occur (AAO, 1996).

Similarly, the American Optometric Association stresses the importance that children receive vision examinations at about <u>6 months</u>, <u>3 years</u> (earlier if abnormalities are detected), and <u>before 1st grade and every 2 years thereafter</u>; more frequent examinations if risk factors are present and based on professional judgment (AOA, 1994).

We can assist in improving early identification of children with vision problems by working together as a team to encourage regular eye examinations with age appropriate tests by pediatricians, family physicians and at school screenings.

For those of you with experience in functional vision assessment and screening, pick and choose what you find useful. This book was written with you in mind, the folks who want a reference to use when doing vision assessments and screenings. So, drop it in your tote bag and off you go. . . .

Kathleen Appleby, M.A.
Educational Vision Consultant

Table of Contents

Introduction Letter 2

Table of Contents 4

BASIC ASSESSMENT INFORMATION 5

Looking At the Visual System in 4 Test Areas 6

Visual Resolution & Health of the Eye 7

Visual Efficiency 8

Visual Perception 9

Visual Pathways 11

PART 1 Vision Assessment of Infants & Children With & Without "Special Needs"
Table of Contents 13

Appendices 71

PART 2 Vision Screening Babies with Play–Table of Contents 93

BASIC ASSESSMENT INFORMATION
THE VISUAL SYSTEM

In order to have a better understanding of vision assessment some background information needs to be laid. It can not be assumed that everyone has the same education in the area of the visual system.

When I began my journey into assessing vision, I saw functional vision assessment as a separate entity and certainly not related to the bigger picture of the visual system. I no longer look at the results in isolation. Dr. Scheiman (1997) looks at the visual system in the Optometric Model of Vision which consists of 3 areas.
1) Acuity, Refractive & Eye Health Disorders.
2) Visual Efficiency Skills.
3) Visual Information Processing Skills.

Dr. Lea Hyvärinen's article, "Assessment of Low Vision in Infants and Children", found on her CD ,"LH-Materials 2001" (available from Vision Associates) discusses the visual system in three parts as follows:

1) Eye and/or anterior visual pathway, (disorders affect quality of the visual image),

2) Pathway between lateral geniculate nucleus (LGN) and/or primary visual cortex (defects that can affect visual fields and cause increased crowding)

3) Cortical or sub-cortical brain functions (disorders of the visual associative cortices are often patchy, affecting specific visual sub-functions.

Dr. Hyvärinen's information is significant in that it offers us understanding of the affects of impairments to brain functions and the performance of the children we service. It can also assist us with setting goals as related to intervention.

Rather than doing vision assessments in rote fashion, it is useful to think of them as avenues to discovery of puzzle pieces used to obtain understanding of the children with whom you work.

I expanded looking at the visual system into 4 test areas. This allowed me to see within which area deficit(s) noted in the assessment fall. It also assisted in determining which "team" member would be the best for referral, based on their expertise and on the child's area of poor performance on the vision assessment

The visual system goes from the front of the eyeball to the visual cortex, so there are many areas of the system to examine when vision deficits are identified or suspected. That's why we need the "team" to take a closer look. A functional vision assessment or a vision screening may identify signs (red flags) that there is something causing a child's performance to deviate from "typical" visual development. This is just the beginning of information gathering. A doctor can then, hopefully, determine the cause of the "red flag".

LOOKING AT THE VISUAL SYSTEM IN 4 TEST AREAS

I find that looking at the visual system in four separate areas of testing beneficial to better understanding a child's overall performance and how it may be impacted by deficits in any of the areas shown in the following chart. Apparent deficiency in one area may find its cause in another. For example, if a child performs poorly on a visual perception test, the cause of the poor performance may be due to visual efficiency deficits. It is important to relate the child's performance in each of the four test areas so the child can be referred to the appropriate specialist.

Eye doctor examinations cover all 4 areas. However, not all eye doctors do so. This is why you need to refer the child to the correct doctor. Ophthalmologists specialize in disease and surgery. Optometrists' training includes emphasis on vision efficiency and vision perception. Vision teachers, school nurses, early intervention staff, therapists, etc. often are responsible to perform functional vision assessments, and vision screenings of some of the domains in the first 3 areas. Since doctors have different specialties, it is important for children to be seen by the appropriate doctor, based on the child's need. Look for a doctor who is good with families, and children with and without special needs. Remind parents they are the consumer and their child's advocate

FOUR VISUAL SYSTEM TEST AREAS

I. RESOLUTION & EYE HEALTH	II. EFFICIENCY	III. PERCEPTION	IV. PATHWAYS
Acuity	Accomodation	Visual Discrimination	Some tests:
Contrast Sensitivity	Binocularity	Visual Figure Gd	VEPM
Visual Fields	Ocular Motility	Visual Closure	CT
Color Vision		Visual Memory	MRI
Adapt Light Change		Visual Spatial Rel	EEG
Amblyopia		Visual Form Cont.	
		Visual Seq Memory	

Vision Associates www.visionkits.com

I. VISUAL RESOLUTION & HEALTH OF THE EYE

It is important for parents to select doctors experienced in the evaluation of infants and children, especially those who have special needs and/or multiple handicaps. The ideal situation is when the parent, teacher and therapist can contribute during the doctor's evaluation. This way functional information can enhance the understanding of how the child uses vision. It can also increase responsiveness of the child during the evaluation.

Evaluations by eye doctors generally cover the following areas with the exception of contrast sensitivity and adaptation to lighting changes. These areas should be measured during routine eye examinations of children with special needs including vision and/or hearing impairments, and adults as well.

Children who have hearing impairments may have unidentified Usher's Syndrome (inherited sensorineural hearing defect and retinitis pigmentosa-inherited retinal degenerations, including visual field loss). This condition may not be known since their high contrast abilities do not initially indicate a visual deficit. The child's decreased ability to adapt to lighting changes and decreases in contrast sensitivity will occur before high contrast acuity is affected. Many programs for the hearing impaired and deaf and blind schools use low contrast tests such as **LEA Symbols Screener** and The **Cone Adaptation to Lighting Changes** to screen for Usher's Syndrome.

VISUAL RESOLUTION AREAS...

Visual Acuity: Measure of eye's ability to distinguish objects details and shape. Problems may affect near or distance acuity.

Ambylopia: Decreased vision in one or both eyes without detectable anatomic damage in eye or visual pathways. Uncorrectable with glasses. It is often referred to as Lazy Eye, however, Dr. Scheiman believes the eye is not really lazy it just has not received proper stimulation for whatever reason.

Contrast Sensitivity: Ability to detect detail having subtle gradations in grayness between test target and background.

Visual Fields: Extent of space visible to an eye as it fixates straight ahead. Measured in degrees away from fixation.

Color Vision: Perception of color, results from stimulation of red (red deficit = protan), green (green deficit = deuteran), and blue cone receptors in retina.

Adaptation to Lighting Changes: When a person with normal vision goes from a lighted area to a low luminance area it takes a few seconds to start seeing colors. In daylight we use cone cells (photopic vision) which inhibit rod cells. When luminance levels decrease, input from cone cells decrease and input from rod cells increase (mesopic vision). When luminance levels decrease further, cone cells contribution to vision stops, colors disappear and the image appears to be in different shades of gray because rod cells do not convey color differences (scotopic vision).

II. VISUAL EFFICIENCY

Dr. Scheiman defines visual efficiency as the effectiveness of the visual system to clearly, efficiently and comfortably allow a person to gather visual information at school or play.

Children with "special needs" are generally seen by pediatric ophthalmologists, a necessary and important part of the "team". Children exhibiting visual efficiency difficulties require additionally important and thorough examinations by optometrists, who specialize in visual function and development (FCOVD or COVD).

"In spite of the significance of visual efficiency problems, they are often undetected even after a professional eye examination. If these problems are suspected, it is incumbent upon an occupational therapist to make a referral to an eye care professional who will perform the type of testing battery that can detect these disorders" (Scheiman, M., 1997).

VISUAL EFFICIENCY AREAS...

Accommodation - Ability to change focus of the eyes so objects at different distances can be seen clearly. It occurs when there is an increase in optical power by the eyes to maintain a clear focus as objects move closer.

Binocularity - The ability to use the two eyes simultaneously and see a single clear image. Influences the ability to localize objects in space accurately and to perceive depth. Lack of binocularity has many causes including: strabismic disorders (eye turn), non-strabismic disorders (includes convergence problems)

Ocular Motility - Eye movements including fixation, saccades (shift of gaze), and ocular pursuits (visually following a moving target).

If a child has a vision problem in the area of visual efficiency it is important to determine if some level of improvement can be achieved, since children with difficulties in these areas frequently exhibit poor school performance and poor visual perception skills. Parents, as consumers and advocates for their children, should select doctors trained in this area who are willing to consult with the family and therapists in reference to activities designed to improve the child's visual efficiency in school and in the home.

III. VISUAL PERCEPTION

One of the most important characteristics of visual perception is that it is organized. We perceive a world of objects, people and events, which move and change in a unified, coherent fashion. Important organizational features of visual perception are the visual constancies, such as brightness, shape and size constancy.

Vision teachers, learning disability teachers, occupational therapists, psychologists & optometrists generally evaluate the following visual perception areas:

Visual Discrimination (VD) - Awareness of distinctive features of forms including shape, orientation, size and color. This is an important skill in reading and math.

Visual Figure-Ground (VFG) - Ability to attend to a specific feature or form while maintaining an awareness of the relationship of this form to background information.

Visual Closure (VC) - Ability to be aware of clues in the visual stimulus that allow determining the final percept with only some of the details present. Visual closure in reading allows us to perceive an entire word accurately when only part of the word is visible.

Visual Memory (VM) - Ability to recognize and recall visually presented information. Spelling requires recall of visual information, reading and math require matching the word/number on the page with a stored image.

Visual Spatial Relationships (VSR) - The ability to develop normal internal and external spatial concepts used to interact with and organize the environment, make judgements about location of objects and the child's body

Visual Form Constancy (VFC) - Ability to recognize that an object has invariant properties such as: shape, position and size even though sensory information received about it has changed. For example, ability to perceiving similarities and differences in geometric figures, symbols, pictures and words.

Visual Sequential Memory (VSM) - Ability to observe, recognize, remember, recall and reproduce the sequence of objects, symbols, etc. in whatever means appropriate for the person.

This book does not discuss ways to formally or informally assess visual perceptual skills. There are standardized tests (motor and non-motor) available to assess these areas. Observations of how children interact with toys and the environment is often the only way to assess visual perception skills in some of the children we service, including babies.

Visual perception is an important part of visual performance and you may wish to include it in your initial assessment. Keep in mind that a child's visual perceptual abilities are no more functional than his or her cognitive abilities (Langley, 1998). I informally observe the child's level of visual perception skills during the vision assessment to gain information on how his or her performance is effected.

GETTING TO "CAUSES" OF VISION PROBLEMS BY IDENTIFICATION OF "SYMPTOMS"...

In my experiences, children with visual deficits in the area of visual efficiency frequently exhibit poor visual perception skills ("symptoms"). It is logical, if poor visual perception skills are assumed, to attempt to remediate them. However, if an eye doctor can determine the "cause" of the vision deficit, and can suggest ways to improve the condition, visual perception remediation may not even be necessary. Remediating visual perception skills when the cause is elsewhere can be unduly frustrating to the child as well as unnecessary.

Assessing visual perception skills of children can be done as pre and post testing after the appropriate doctor determines:

- The "cause" of the vision problem (get to the "cause"),
- If there is something that can be done to improve the child's visual condition (treat the "cause", not the "symptom").
- The potential for improvement of the visual condition,
- The approach to obtain the improvement.

Keep in mind that a child may exhibit poor visual perception skills based on deficits in visual efficiency. If there is nothing that can be done to improve the situation then it will be necessary to develop compensation and remediation goals, as the child's performance is partly reflective of his or her perceptions. In addition, some children may have poor visual perception function, or lack of function due to brain damage. Functional assessment of perception is necessary to plan goals for these children.

IV. VISUAL PATHWAYS

"A vision problem could still be present even if an individual has good visual acuity, no refractive error or eye health disorder and has normal accommodation, binocular vision and ocular motility. Vision is more than just seeing clearly and comfortably. An individual must also be able to analyze, interpret and make use of the incoming visual information in order to interact with the environment" (Scheiman, M., 1994).

Deficits in the visual pathways and the location of lesions are critical to better understanding what meaning a child might be able to derive from what his or her eyes take in. Medical doctors test this area of the visual system with a variety of tests, including but not limited to:

Visual Evoked Potential Map (VEP) = a form of computerized Encephalogram (EEG) and can detect processing or lack thereof and visual stimuli by the visual cortex.

Computerized Tomography (CT) or **Magnetic Resonance Imaging** (MRI)

Encephalogram (EEG) = measures electrical activity of the brain and can provide information about the functioning of the occipital cortex.

Dr. Hyvärinen, on her CD, "LH-Materials 2001", presents us with excellent information, including the following list of disorders of visual functions that may be the result of lesions on certain visual pathways..

VISUAL SUB-FUNCTIONS POSSIBLY AFFECTED BY DISORDERS OF CORTICAL/SUBCORTICAL BRAIN FUNCTIONS...

Recognition of persons by facial features,

Recognition of facial expressions,

Perception of objects on a patterned background,

Perception of size or directions,

Eye-hand coordination,

Orientation in egocentric and allocentric space,

Evaluation of surface qualities,

Place, movement and/or speed of objects.

This information is quite fascinating and, hopefully, someday will be consistently covered in vision assessments utilizing proper tests and materials. We can include the above in our observations of the child, whenever possible. As we start to look at how the brain functions in relationship to the child's performance we will get insight into the benefits of certain intervention approaches, albeit, in some cases, trial and error.

Once tests are developed we will be better equipped to decide if certain repetition of some activities and stimuli are really necessary or even appropriate. Wouldn't it be wonderful to develop intervention goals based more frequently on brain function versus based on trial and error? The times they are "a-changin" and as we learn more so will our work with children change.

VISION ASSESSMENT
of Infants & Children with & w/o Special Needs

by Kathleen Appleby, MA

PART I

Vision Assessment of Infants & Special Needs Children

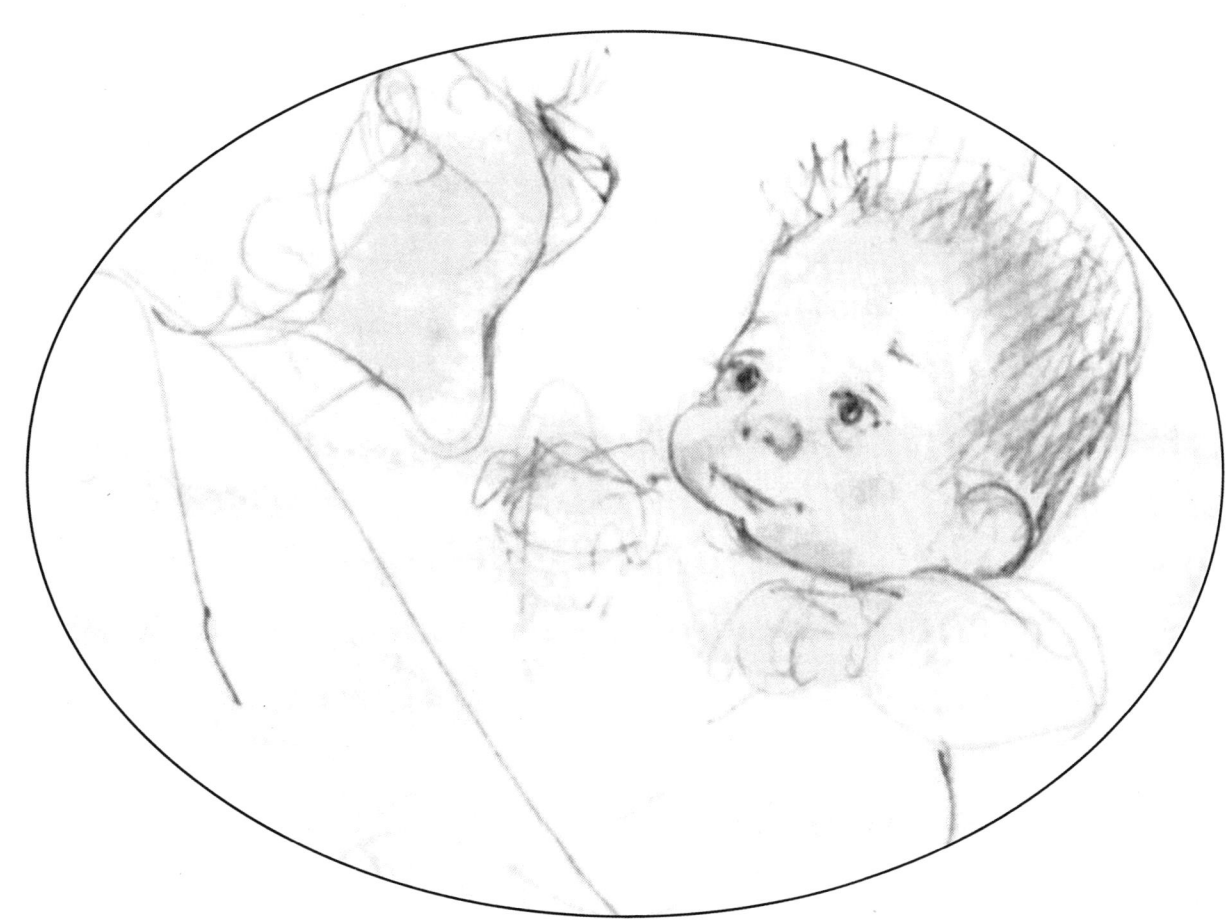

TABLE OF CONTENTS

PART 1
VISION ASSESSMENT OF INFANTS & SPECIAL NEEDS CHILDREN

Table of Contents 15

Greetings Again 16

Typical Visual Development 17

Cortical/Cerebral Visual Impairments (C/CVI) 19

Before Assessing Vision 25

Importance of Sequencing the Assessment 28

VISION ASSESSMENT PROCEDURE

Let's Begin: Pretend You Are a "Sleuth" 31
Observation & Interview 32
Pupillary Response 34
Visual Sphere/Visual Awareness 36
Fixation 39
Muscle Balance 41
Visually Following Moving Toy/Ocular Pursuits 44
Movement of Both Eyes Inward/Convergence 46
Shift of Gaze/Saccades 48
Visual Fields 51
Acuity: Functional, Grating, Optotype 53
Contrast Sensitivity 60
Suppression 63
Stereopsis 65
Color Vision 67
Vision Perception 69

APPENDIX (page 71)
Scope & Sequence: Vision Assessment Tests & Materials .... A
FORM: Parent/Care Taker Interview .... B
FORM: Typical Visual Development C
CHECKLIST: Characteristics of Cerebral Visual Impairment .... D
FORMS: Recording .... E
FORMS: Reporting .... F
REFERENCES: Cortical/Cerebral Visual Impairment .... G
BIBLIOGRAPHY/REFERENCES .... H

Greetings again,

Now we're almost ready to branch off into the "step by step" guide for each of the vision assessment areas covered in this book. However, before we do so we need to gather some more information.

First of all we need to gather information about the child from the parents or care givers (see Interview Form in Appendix A). We also need to gather information about the child through checklists completed by parents and those other important people in the child's life. In addition don't forget to become familiar with the child's medical history. Forms to assist you can be found in the Appendix.

Second we need to review the chart listing the visual development of "typically" developing children. This is important so you know when there are deviations in the child's visual development. This indicates the child may have a vision problem.

And finally, you will learn about Cortical/Cerebral Vision Impairment and how damage to the brain can affect visual function. This is so important because you need to use different assessment techniques with these children.

Keep in mind that vision assessments and vision screenings do not replace evaluations by eye doctors. Many non-visual factors can effect performance, such as motor abilities, processing skills, cooperation and cognitive abilities.

What is covered in this book is not necessarily a representation of a true "functional" vision assessment, as functional refers to assessing vision as the child performs "functional" daily tasks and interactions with his or her environment. In addition to observations and some structured activities, actual tests are used in more diagnostic ways. Look at the information in this book as a way to assess vision including "functional" components.

"It takes a team to assess for vision problems" and you are part of that team. It takes doctors, parents/family, teachers, therapists and the child to round out the information needed. Don't be shy about asking members on the team for the information you need and about sharing the information you obtain from vision assessments and vision screenings. Children are part of the "team" because they are our best teachers. By observing them closely you will see what I mean; no vision assessment is complete without observation.

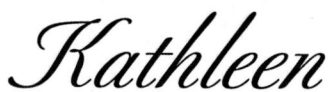

"TYPICAL" VISUAL DEVELOPMENT

In order to assess vision you will need to review visual development of children who are developing typically so you can identify deviations from typical development. The following chart can be used as a guide. In some cases you may not be looking for deviations but for any signs of vision.

VISUAL DEVELOPMENT OF "TYPICALLY" DEVELOPING CHILDREN

AGE   **BEHAVIOR**

Birth - 1 month
- __Turns eyes & head to look at light sources
- __Appears to look through rather than at people
- __Black & white (high contrast) objects most interesting
- __PUPILS RESPOND TO LIGHT may be constricted 1st few weeks
- __FIXATION noted as child nurses with open eyes
- __MUSCLE BALANCE eye turn may be present, aligning later
- __HORIZONTAL PURSUITS with head movement, may be jerky
- __VERTICAL PURSUITS emerging
- __SHIFT OF GAZE from toy to toy slow with head movement
- __ACUITY poor due to immaturity of retina
- __CONTRAST SENSITIVITY poor due to immaturity of retina

2-3 months
- __Social smile by 3 months
- __Reaches toward & later grasps hanging objects.
- __FIXATION intense eye contact, interest in looking at moving lips
- __VERTICAL/HORIZONTAL PURSUITS with eyes only.
- __PERIPHERAL VISUAL RESPONSES within 60°
- __COLOR VISION prefers colored toys to black & white
- __ACCOMMODATES to different distances by 3 months
- __STEREOPSIS by 3 months

4 - 6 months
- __First time watching own hands is noted
- __Reaches toward faces & objects
- __Watches toys fall or roll away
- __VISUAL SPHERE gradually extends outward
- __SHIFT OF GAZE across midline
- __CONVERGENCE present by 6 months
- __PERIPHERAL VISUAL FIELDS responses within 180°
- __ACUITY recognizes distance objects, watches his or her hands.

7-10 months
- __Interest in pictures in books
- __Recognizes partially hidden objects
- __Pictures in books become interesting
- __FIXATION eye hand coordination improving
- __PERIPHERAL VISION symmetrical
- __ACUITY notices small objects like cereal & crumbs
- __PERCEPTION develops perception to form & size

11-12 months
- __Looks through window
- __Recognizes people, objects and pictures
- __Likes to play Peek-a-book
- __DEPTH PERCEPTION explores depth by looking into containers
- __COLOR PERCEPTION full color vision.

Vision Associates www.visionkits.com

WHAT A ONE YEAR OLD WITH "TYPICAL" VISUAL DEVELOPMENT SHOULD BE ABLE TO DO...

Accurately fixate without eye or head turn,

Smoothly shift gaze across midline,

Smoothly converge eyes to 3" from the nose.

Smoothly follow moving toys horizontally & vertically with eye movement and without head movement.

Visually accommodate, focus on objects at different distances.

Upper visual fields reaching adult size and horizontal and lower fields smaller than adult size (Mohn & Hof-van-Duin, 1986)

Acuity continues to improve as the retina matures.

Contrast sensitivity reaching adult levels at about 3 years of age. (Hyvärinen, 1988).

SPOTTING BABIES WITH "NON-TYPICAL" VISUAL DEVELOPMENT...

The following list will assist you in spotting babies who may have deficits in visual development so you can quickly refer the family to a pediatric ophthalmologist.

Signs during infancy that may indicate a vision problem

Lack of visual fixation of following by 3 months.

Lack of accurate reaching for objects by 6 months.

Persistent lack of the eyes moving in concert or the sustained "crossing" of one eye after about 4-6 months.

Frequent horizontal or vertical jerky eye movements (nystagmus).

Lack of a clear, black pupil (eg, haziness of the cornea, a whitish appearance inside the pupil, or a significant asymmetry of the usual "red eye" appearance of a flash photograph).

Persistent tearing when the infant is not crying.

Significant sensitivity to bright light (photophobia).

Persistent redness of the normally white conjunctiva,

Drooping of an eyelid sufficient to obscure the pupil,

Any asymmetry of pupillary size,

CORTICAL/CEREBRAL VISUAL IMPAIRMENTS

When assessing vision it is important be aware that there are children who have vision deficits that are due to ocular impairment and children who have vision deficits based on Cortical/Cerebral visual impairment, or a combination of both.

WHAT IS AN OCULAR IMPAIRMENT?...

An ocular impairment includes deficits anywhere from/and including the eyeball through the anterior visual pathways (from the retina to the lateral geniculate body).

WHAT IS A CORTICAL/CEREBRAL VISUAL IMPAIRMENT (C/CVI)?

Dr. James Jan explains in his article, "Visual Behaviors and Adaptations Associated with Cortical and Ocular Impairment in Children", that lesions on the posterior visual pathway from the lateral geniculate body to the visual cortex can cause cortical visual loss. Damage can occur either before or after birth. He goes on to state that although damage to almost any part of the brain can cause changes in visual behaviors and perception, only damage to the posterior visual pathways, including the visual cortex can cause cortical visual loss.

Dr. Lea Hyvärinen suggests using "cerebral" rather than "cortical" visual disability or "cerebral visual disturbance" since often both cortical and sub-cortical visual functions may be involved rather than only cortical functions.

Be sure to check out the references and read, read, read especially Dr. James Jan's articles about cortical visual impairment. I have found his research extremely informative and an excellent reference when assessing and working with children with cortical/cerebral visual impairments (C/CVI). See the C/CVI Reference list for further reading, as this is an area that requires further sturdy.

Dr. Hyvärinen's teachings on brain damage is absolutely necessary to better understand how certain damaged areas affect visual function. Her CD, "LH-Materials 2001", available from Vision Associates, is an excellent teaching tool. The CD provides more detail, including videos of children with various visual limitations being tested.

THE IMPORTANCE OF TIMELY DIAGNOSIS OF C/CVI FOR CRITICAL AND EARLY INTERVENTION...

Early vision intervention is critical for children with Cerebral Visual Impairments (C/CVI), as documented in the research and explained in the following references. A child may be suspected of having a cerebral visual loss when the extent of visual loss is unexplained by ocular abnormalities. Services from a teacher of the Visually Impaired generally require a doctor's report stating that cerebral visual impairment is suspected based on the child's history, functional performance, and behavior characteristics. Some children with C/CVI may also have ocular abnormalities.

WHY DIAGNOSE C/CVI QUICKLY?...

Dr. Jan and co-authors (1985) explain why. "...cerebral insult can produce coexisting damage to the eyes and visual cortex, but cortical visual loss is rarely diagnosed (if ever) in these children, yet the correct diagnosis would make a major difference in their visual rehabilitation."

"Because CVI is a hidden handicap, the children are frequently described as visually inattentive or poorly motivated. A great number of neurological disorders can cause CVI, but after the initial insult to the brain, vision tends to improve in the majority of children. Those whose vision does not improve 1-1/2 to 2 years after the onset of their cortical visual loss are less likely to improve" Jan, J., (1990).

"Children with CVI and ocular visual loss radically differ in their ability to process visual messages. With ocular disorders, the signals may be incomplete, but the process of analysis is sound. Thus, visual enrichment and training in scanning more efficiently when the information is complex are successful techniques. For children with CVI, this approach does not work; in fact, visual input must be controlled to avoid "visual overloading"...if the amount of visual information is increased, it becomes much more difficult for the children to process visual input. Visual images should be simple in form and presented in isolation" Jan, J., (1990).

ETIOLOGY OF PERMANENT CEREBRAL VISUAL IMPAIRMENT...

<u>Prenatal</u> (before birth)
Toxemia, Intra-Uterine Infection, Cerebral Dysgenesis

<u>Perinatal</u> (birth to 28 days of life)
Asphyxia, Intra-Cerebral Hemorrhage, Meningitis/Encephalitis

<u>Acquired</u>
Shunt malfunction, Trauma, Meningitis, Cortical Vein Thrombosis, Cardiac Arrest, Shaken Baby Syndrome

CHARACTERISTICS OF CEREBRAL VISUAL IMPAIRMENT CHECKLIST

Children with other types of visual impairments may exhibit some of these characteristics. Please check any areas below that pertain to the child.

APPEARANCE

___Does not look blind
___Blank facial expression
___Lack of visual communication skills
___Eye movements smooth, but aimless
___Nystagmus (rapid eye movement) rarely seen

VISION FUNCTION

___Visual function varies from day to day or hour to hour
___Limited visual attention and lacks visual curiosity
___Aware of distant objects, but not able to identify
___Spontaneous visual activity has short duration
___Visual learning tiring
___Closes eyes while listening
___Balance improved with eyes closed
___Look away from people and objects
___Consistently look to either side when visual looking
___When visually reaching looks with a slight downward gaze
___Turns head to side when reaching, as if using peripheral fields
___Uses touch to identify objects

MOBILITY SKILLS

___Occasionally "sees" better traveling in a car
___Difficulties with depth perception, inaccurate reach
___Unable to estimate distances
___Difficulties with spatial interpretation
___Avoids obstacles, but unable to use vision for close work

IMPROVED VISUAL PERFORMANCE

___When in familiar environments and when using familiar objects
___When told "what" to look for and "where" to look
___When objects are held close to eyes when viewing
___When objects are widely spaced
___When looking at one object verses a group of objects
___When color is used to assist in identification of objects or shapes
___When objects are against a plain background & paired with movement & sound

Adapted: Jan, J., Groenveld, A., Sykanda, A., Hoyt, C. (1987)

UNDERSTANDING BEHAVIORS AS THEY RELATE TO VISION IN THE CHILD WITH C/CVI...

Children with C/CVI respond differently as related to amounts & locations of damage in the posterior areas of their visual systems. Some children may also have ocular impairments.

FLUCTUATING VISUAL RESPONSIVENESS INCLUDING

- ❏ The level of visual awareness changes
- ❏ Days when child appears not to see
- ❏ Usual refocusing techniques do not necessarily work

MANY EXTERNAL CONDITIONS AFFECT VISUAL ATTENTION

- ❏ Noisy environments
- ❏ Confused by choice of activities needing refocusing
- ❏ Sick or tired
- ❏ Medication

LACK OF VISUAL ATTENTION & SPONTANEITY RELATE TO

- ❏ Difficulty with object recognition
- ❏ Depth perception limitations
- ❏ Poor concepts of space & distance

UNUSUAL LOOKING BEHAVIORS

- ❏ Self stimulation
- ❏ Eye pressing is unusual
- ❏ Flicking fingers in front of light source seen occasionally
- ❏ Light gazing most often seen when no usable vision
- ❏ Children with usable vision light gaze but not obsessively
- ❏ Does not look blind
- ❏ Nystagmus absent unless additional ocular impairments
- ❏ Fixation & visual pursuits may occur fleetingly
- ❏ Eye movements smooth but aimless
- ❏ Look away from people or tasks\ or when reaching

INTERVENTION SUGGESTIONS FOR CHILDREN WITH CORTICAL/CEREBRAL VISION IMPAIRMENT

It is important to note that children who have C/CVI need different intervention approaches than children who have ocular type impairments. There is no "cookbook" approach to selecting the most appropriate visual activities for children but often children with diminished vision, based on ocular deficits, respond positively to heightened visual stimulation in the beginning stages of visual responsiveness. However, the approach with children with C/CVI is different. Use the suggestions below as they pertain to the child.

SUGGESTIONS TO ASSIST INTERACTIONS WITH CHILDREN WITH C/CVI

Every child is different when it comes to developing a plan for intervention and integration of vision into his or her daily life. All aspects of the child must be taken into consideration,e.g., motor, communication, cognition, physical health, environmental, processing. All suggestions need to be adapted to the child's developmental level.

Strategies that appear appropriate can be utilized in a "trial and error" fashion with the child. If they result in improved visual responses and over all interactions with the child repeat the strategies. Be aware of signs of improvement in the child's levels of performance so you can phase out adaptations to encourage more realistic presentations. Avoid isolated activities that do not have real life carryover whenever appropriate and possible. Encourage utilization of the strategies during daily activities so the child becomes more "functionally" visual.

Levels: Take the child's motor, cognitive and communication levels into consideration and present activities adapted to these levels.

Avoid Visual Clutter: Present objects against a plain background & widely spaced. Some children may have difficulty visually discriminating objects from the background. Some children may have to close their eyes to control over stimulation. Some children hold objects close to their eyes to fill the entire visual fields and eliminate visual distraction.

Pair the Object: Use sound, movement, color &/or a child's touch paired with the object. Some C/CVI children visually respond best to movement of objects, usually in their periphery. Use simple descriptions of "what" the object is and "where" the object is located, etc. For example, "Look at your cup. It is on the table." Use touch cautiously since some children are tactilly defensive and this may be upsetting.

Perception of Object: Encourage the child to experience the object in as many ways as possible so he/she can develop the "ness" of the object. For example, give the child opportunities to hold, peel, smell, cut and eat a banana. This will assist in the development of the perception of "banana" so the child can better understand what is seen. The child may have "piecemeal" vision and have difficulty perceiving the total "image" of objects. Utilize techniques used for a blind child by introducing new objects, encouraging tactile exploration of the entire object.

Visual Gaze: Peripheral gaze may be necessary verses a direct central gaze, i.e., the child may look at the object and then look away when reaching. It may be that the child is only able to integrate one sensory input at a time or he or she may be using peripheral vision.

Visual Preferences: Determine the child's preference for objects by size and color. Place these objects in the location that the child most frequently looks toward while the child is in his or her most stable and comfortable position.

Environment: Be sensitive to the child's surroundings and time of day. Adapt the surroundings to reduce noise, clutter, glare, etc. For example, I place a plain sheet over the furniture when working on the floor in a child's home. I also wear a plain light colored apron to present objects against.

Objects: Use real & familiar objects verse abstract objects, i.e., teach "attributes", "same & different" and "visual discrimination" by sorting spoons & forks vs. circles and squares, etc., when appropriate. Children with C/CVI typically have difficulty generalizing between objects, i.e., they may know their own cup but can may not know a different looking cup is also a cup. Keep the objects and placements constant initially until the concept is established then broaden the activity to include similar objects.

Active Learning: Engage the child in a play situation at his/her levels and encourage independent interactions to avoid passive learning. Utilize a routine/pattern of interaction and repetition. Empathize a clear beginning and end to activities. Work on a tray when possible to offer a space within which to present materials. Offer adequate time and cueing when there is a transition between activities. Use short "working" sessions.

Communication: Utilize a "calendar box", when appropriate, to offer a clear beginning and end to activities. A "calendar box", based on Dr. Van Dijk's theories, consists of small boxes placed side by side with real objects, one object per box, velcroed on the boxes. Each object provides a tactile representation of each of the child's daily activities, The teacher talks to the child about the sequence of the day as he or she looks at and feels each of the objects. Later the child looks at and feels the object before each activity and takes it off the box and puts it in the box when the activity is over and then goes on to the next box to find the object representing the next activity. For example, use an empty juice box to represent snack time. Phase the objects to symbolic representations of the object when the child is able to generalize the meaning, i.e., replace the juice carton (representing snack) with a straw.

BEFORE ASSESSING FUNCTIONAL VISION

BEFORE ASSESSING BABIES &/or CHILDREN WITH SPECIAL NEEDS: THINK ABOUT <u>WHY</u> YOU ARE ASSESSING...

Babies who have serious, unidentified, vision impairments will have delays in their visual and general development and may not be aware of vision for a long time. Vision is an excellent activator of brain function so visual stimulation and multi-modality stimulation may be necessary to stimulate baby's awareness of vision. Vision stimulation strengthens and activates synapses in the brain. Synapses that are not used will wither away in a process called pruning (Begley, 1997).

SOME <u>REASONS</u> TO ASSESS VISION...

- ❏ Gathering information to share with the doctor for in depth evaluation.
- ❏ Determine areas of limited visual performance needing intervention/stimulation.
- ❏ Discovering the levels of residual vision.
- ❏ Determining what adaptations are necessary.
- ❏ Determining intervention and compensation strategies.
- ❏ To determine changes to functional vision as ongoing part of the child's program.

BEFORE ASSESSING TAKE INTO <u>CONSIDERATION</u>...

- ❏ Child's age, handicaps and levels of functioning as these areas can have implications to the assessment outcomes.
- ❏ If the baby is premature, use adjusted age to compare with the expected ranges.
- ❏ A baby's or a multiple handicapped child's response patterns of breathing, quieting, smiling, babbling. This assists in detecting visual reactions to your toys.
- ❏ Allow adequate response time. A multiple handicapped child may be slow to respond.
- ❏ Medical conditions, such as infants with severe visual impairment, Retinopathy of Prematurity (ROP), and after recent eye surgery, may have difficulty detecting stationary objects.

- Mode of communication: gesturing, eye gaze, etc. This is where interviews with family and school staff can be of great importance.

- Medications and seizure history.

- Environment: Is it too noisy, distracting?

- Positioning: determine the best position for the best visual responses to complete the assessment. In addition repeat some of the assessment tasks with the child in his or her usual body and head position, even if it is not conducive to the best visual responses. Be prepared to discuss both performance levels to contrast the differences in visual responses.

KEEP THESE TIPS IN MIND...

- Use the child's own toy as a "looking motivator" if there is no interest in your toys.

- Position the child so his/her body & head are supported

- If possible choose the time of day the child is most alert and relaxed.

- Use a play situation to familiarize the child with preferential looking testing.

- Premature babies and multiple handicapped children are easily over stimulated so watch closely for signs of over stimulation and give them frequent rest periods.

- Wear plain clothes to provide contrast to assessment objects and to make viewing easier for children who may be overwhelmed by too much visual information

- Position the child so he/she faces you. and away from windows and busy background You may need to lay the child on the floor and lean over him or her or lay on the floor next to the child.

- The baby can look over the parent's shoulder while being held, sit in the parent's lap, or sit in his/her chair.

- Consider the child's most comfortable position and support his/her head so involuntary motor movements least affect visual performance.

- Plan your time, it may take several visits with the child to complete the assessment.

WHEN ASSESSING CHILDREN WITH CORTICAL/CEREBRAL VISUAL IMPAIRMENTS (C/CVI) INCLUDE THESE SUGGESTIONS...

- ❑ Look at the medical and birth history of the child before assessing the child. Review the differences between ocular and cortical/cerebral vision impairment in reference to assessment techniques. Take the time to learn as much as you can about cortical/cerebral visual impairments., as well as other medical conditions.

- ❑ If a central presentation does not elicit a visual response, try moving the object in the periphery.

- ❑ Utilize objects they are interested in or familiar with to elicit a visual response.

- ❑ Simplify the presentation.

- ❑ Wear plain clothes.

VISION INFORMATION TO SHARE WITH THE DOCTOR...

Long and detailed reports are fine and appreciated by teachers, therapists and parents, but doctors need short, condensed, informational one page summaries including responses that are important to share:

- ❑ Family history of vision problems.

- ❑ Latency of eye movements when following moving targets

- ❑ Unusual eye movements

- ❑ Unusual head positions

- ❑ Unusual fixation, such as, looking through a person or avoiding looking

- ❑ Small fixation jerks until gaze reaches target rather than one smooth shift of gaze.

- ❑ Describe the conditions in which you get the best and poorest visual responses.

- ❑ Describe the conditions in which you got no visual responses.

- ❑ Eye pressing

- ❑ Roving eye movements

- ❑ Nystagmus (rapid eye movement)

- ❑ Light gazing

- ❑ Any unusual visual responses

IMPORTANCE OF SEQUENCING THE ASSESSMENT

"Vision is critical to all areas of development and learning. Moreover, the effective and efficient use of vision, including visual function and visual perception, is learned and follows a developmental progression." Zambone A.M. (1989).

Visual assessment of infants and children with multihandicaps is best completed in sequence. Quality tests are now available that support comprehensive assessment. Results of the assessment can be combined with the visual information obtained in ongoing observation of children as they are engaged in everyday activities. (Hyvärinen, L. 1994)

Vision Assessment Sequence	Birth-3 Yrs Assessment	Sp Needs Assessment	Baby Screen	Play Screen	Pre School Screen
Observation & Interview	X	X	X	X	X
Pupillary Responses	X	X	X	X	
Visual Sphere/Attention	X	X	X	X	
Fixation	X	X	X	X	X
Muscle Balance	X	X	X	X	X
Ocular Pursuits	X	X	X	X	X
Convergence	X	X	X	X	X
Shift of Gaze	X	X	X	X	X
Visual Fields	X	X	X	X	X
Acuity Functional	X	X	X	X	
Acuity Gratings	X	X	X		
Acuity Optotypes		X		X	X
Contrast Sensitivity	X	X	X		X
Suppression/Binocularity				X	X
Stereopsis/Depth	X	X			X
Color Vision				X	X
Vision Perception	Full Assess	Full Assess			Full Assess
"Vis Assess of Inf & Chn.."	PART 1	PART 1	PART 2	PART 2	

SUGGESTED SEQUENCE OF A VISION ASSESSMENT

Utilize play situations and follow the suggested sequence, whenever possible, as some visual areas build on the next area. For example, visual sphere should be completed before fixation because a lack of fixation may be due to being out of the child's visual sphere. You will probably not always be able to assess all the listed areas, but do so when possible.

Often times a child's responses will guide the direction of the assessment, so, follow the child's lead and curiosity and when appropriate, deviate from the sequence. This is similar to a "teachable moment". Be sure to take the time to get familiar with the child and with his and her response patterns and give the child time to get use to you, develop rapport and use a playful situation to do the assessment.

WHAT YOU'LL FIND IN EACH AREA OF A FUNCTIONAL VISION ASSESSMENT...

EXPECTED OUTCOMES WHEN COMPARED TO "TYPICAL" VISUAL DEVELOPMENT... from children who follow "typical" visual development.

PROCEDURES to follow to assess each area of the assessment.

BE CONCERNED IF... a list of responses to watch for that indicate possible vision problems.

BE PLEASED IF... any visual responses are noted in children who do not generally react visually.

VISION ASSESSMENT PROCEDURE

LET'S BEGIN: PRETEND YOU ARE A "SLEUTH"

Think of yourself as a detective solving the mysteries of where possible causes of vision problems occur. Even though it is advisable to follow a suggested testing sequence the child may lead the "assessment dance" based on a variety of things, such as, the child's interest, the need for a quick look at a skill and/or the toy/penlight already in your hand. However, the child's responses, or lack of, may direct your next interaction.

It is important that you maintain focus on why your are testing and how you intend to test, based on the child's needs. Planning your time is also important. It may take several sessions to complete the assessment. You can use the recording and reporting forms found in the Appendix.

The child's responses should inspire you to ask yourself questions. For example, if the child fixates at a wildly interesting toy with a head turn or with an unusual eye position you should be forming questions in your mind as to why the unusual response occurred.

I like to pretend I am the child I'm assessing, sitting in that wheel chair or being held in mom's arms. Look at what the child is facing toward. A window or a visually overstimulating wall? Turn the child so that he/she faces a plain plain background. What does the child's body position tell me. Remember it is not only visual responses we are looking for; we learn a lot about what is too visually stimulating to a child when he or she consistently avoids looking.

Ask yourself questions such as, "Why did the child turn his/her head to fixate? Was it because of poorer acuity in the non-fixation eye than in the fixing eye. Was the child using eccentric fixation (fixating off the macula/fovea, best area to see on the retina)? Could the eye turn be caused by a muscle imbalance or a visual field deficit? Thus, you may wish to go to the area you suspect next to check out your hunch. Playing detective will serve you well, as children are our best teachers and guides; don't miss an opportunity. Your observations will give you valuable information to share with the "team".

In order to get a response or decrease visual distractions you may need to wiggle objects, move them closer or place them in front of a plain background. If there is still no response move the objects slowly in the child's periphery, alternating sides to determine if the child responds only to one side. Air movement can cause a reaction not visually initiated, so take care not to cause air movement.

If there is no response at the usual luminance level to any of your objects, even at close distance, try lower and higher luminance levels. If no response is seen try a light box and illuminated toys at low luminance levels to increase contrast. Be aware of the possibility that there might be vision only in some extreme corner of the visual field, thus an unusual head position may be noted. Now let's begin . . .

OBSERVATION & INTERVIEW

Interpretation of a child's functional vision is more than the sum of the components of a vision assessment. That is why it is important to observe the child during everyday activities to get insights into his or her use of vision. In addition some children may over react to stimulation. Relaxation techniques may be necessary to get the best visual responses. Close observation of the child & consultation with other "team" members can assist in this important area. It's important to compare the child's responses in two situations: the child's "real life" and "ideal" situation as it relates to visual responses.

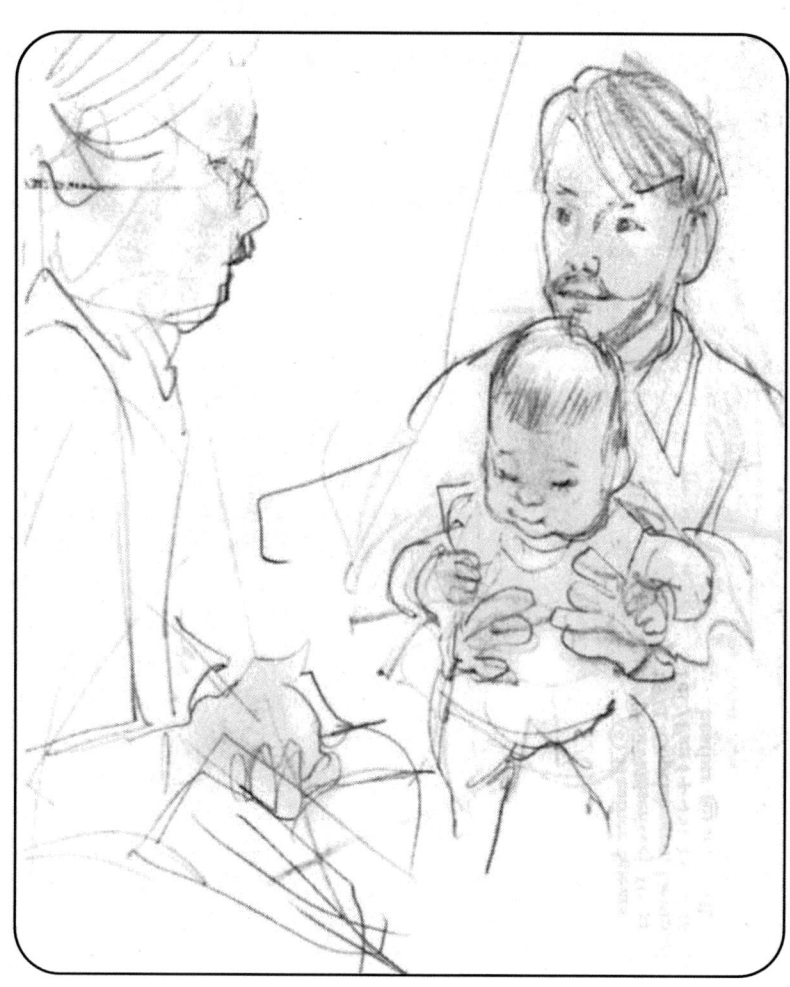

EXPECTED OUTCOMES WHEN COMPARED TO "TYPICAL" VISUAL DEVELOPMENT...

No unusual behaviors should be noted such as head turn or tilt, unusual eye turn, unusual or lack of fixation, eye poking, lack of visual communication, aimless eye movement, or nystagmus (rapid eye movement), i.e. In children who generally exhibit no visual responses, any visual responses are important to note.

PROCEDURE...

1) Utilizing any stimulus, familiarize yourself with child's response patterns, such as: Breathing Changes, Quieting, Eye Widening, Smiling, Babbling, or Reaching for toy.

2) If you observe any of these responses when presenting the child with a visually stimulating toy, it is possible that he/she is exhibiting visual awareness to the toy even though you might not see fixation.

3) If the child does not appear to fixate on the object look for the presence of any of the response patterns in #1.

4) Position the child so he/she faces the examiner. Consider his or her most comfortable position and support his/her head so involuntary motor movements least affect his/her visual performance.

5) Child can look over the parent's shoulder while being held, sit in their lap, or sit in his/her chair, if appropriate.

6) Allow adequate response time when making observations. Multiple handicapped children need extended time.

7) Adapt the procedures to the child's developmental levels.

8) Present the child with a visually stimulating toy, not paired with sound or movement, unless necessary to elicit a visual response.

9) Be cautious when using moving striped materials or when using flickering lights with seizure prone children.

BE CONCERNED IF...

- ❏ Child lacks interest in looking, avoids fixation, tends to look away from people and things
- ❏ Visual responses fluctuate day to day
- ❏ Smooth but aimless eye movements
- ❏ Closes an eye when looking
- ❏ Eye or head turn
- ❏ Excessive blinking or squints
- ❏ Eye pressing
- ❏ Horizontal or vertical jerky rapid eye movements (nystagmus)
- ❏ Light gazing
- ❏ Lack of accurate reaching by 6 months
- ❏ Persistent tearing when not crying
- ❏ Any unusual appearance of the eyes, e.g., cloudy lenses

BE PLEASED IF...

No unusual responses are noted.
Visual responses are noted in children who do not generally react visually.

PUPILLARY RESPONSES TO LIGHT

Have you ever wondered why you should look at pupillary responses when assessing a child's vision? One important reason is to observe any unusual responses that may indicate a change from the responses noted by the eye doctor, indicating possible visual changes. If that is the situation inform the parent/s so they can share the information with the doctor.

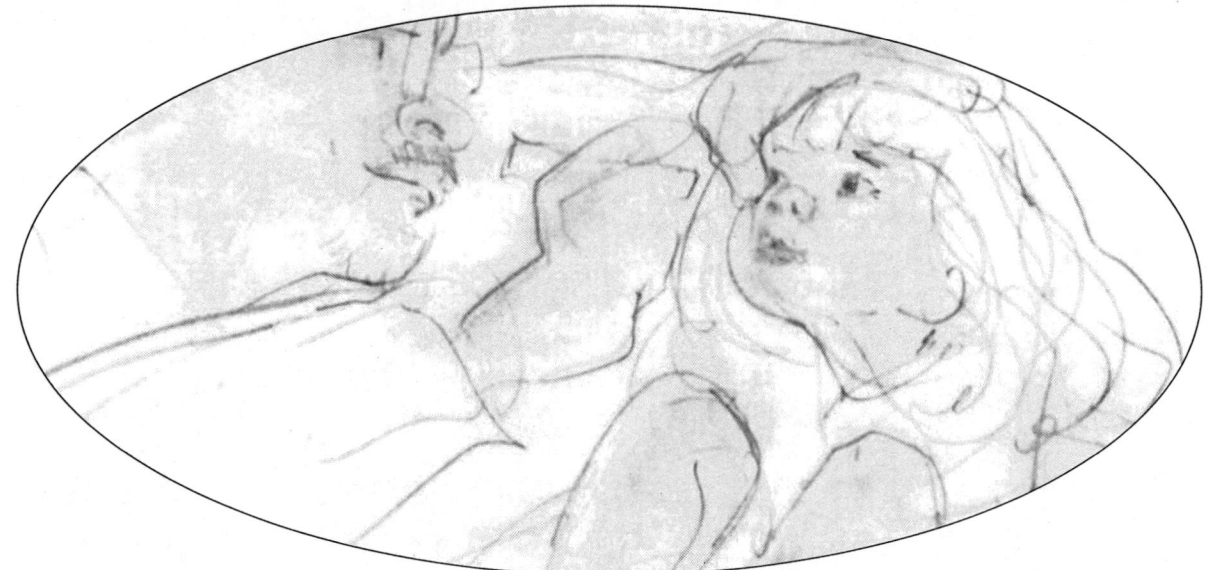

When observing pupillary responses keep in mind that it is reported that infant's pupils tend to be smaller than when 12 months of age (Riordan-Eva, 1989). Infants with dark eyes tend to have smaller pupillary diameters than do infants with lighter irides (Martin, 1989). Infant's pupil sizes also vary from baby to baby. Pupillary responses are subcortical. The state of alertness, attentiveness and reactions to medications can influence pupil size. Some eye conditions are related to the iris, such as aniridia (absence of some of the iris), iris coloboma (failure of the fetal fissure to close in early embryonic life with a 'keyhole' defect with no effect on vision).and other pupillary anomalies. This makes observing pupillary responses difficult in infants.

EXPECTED OUTCOMES WHEN COMPARED TO "TYPICAL" VISUAL DEVELOPMENT...
Normal pupillary responses include pupils constricting in bright light and dilating in dim light.

Both pupils should constrict equally and be the same size when a penlight is held between the eyes at 18".

When you hold the edge of your hand on the child's nose to block the light of the penlight from one eye and briefly shine the penlight in the eye opposite the light, and that pupil also constricts.

Keep in mind a responsive pupil does not necessarily imply a child's visual system is intact.

PROCEDURE:
Do not assess pupillary responses if the child is medically involved, seizure prone or on medication.

1) Place the child in the best position for comfort and motor stability and head control.

2) If the pupils do not constrict in bright light do not assess this area and advise the parent to protect the child's eyes and inform the eye doctor.

3) Dim the lights in the room and after a short while turn the lights on and observe the child's eyes.

4) Maintain dim light for the following activities.

5) Use a penlight and hold it about 18" from the child's nose and turn it on. Both pupils should constrict equally and be the same size. (Direct)

6) Hold the edge of your hand between each eye to separate the light between eyes.

7) Quickly shine the penlight in the right eye and watch the response in the left eye.

8) Repeat on the other side. The eye opposite from the light should constrict too (consensual).

BE CONCERNED IF...
- ❏ The pupils do not get smaller (constrict) in reaction to the light.
- ❏ Each pupil is a different size during the _accommodative_ procedure.
- ❏ Each pupil is a different size in average room lighting.
- ❏ During the _consensual_ task the eye that _does not_ have a light in it does not get smaller.
- ❏ There is no pupillary response to the light.
- ❏ Lack of a clear, black pupil

BE PLEASED IF...
The pupils react as expected in "typical" visual development.

VISUAL SPHERE

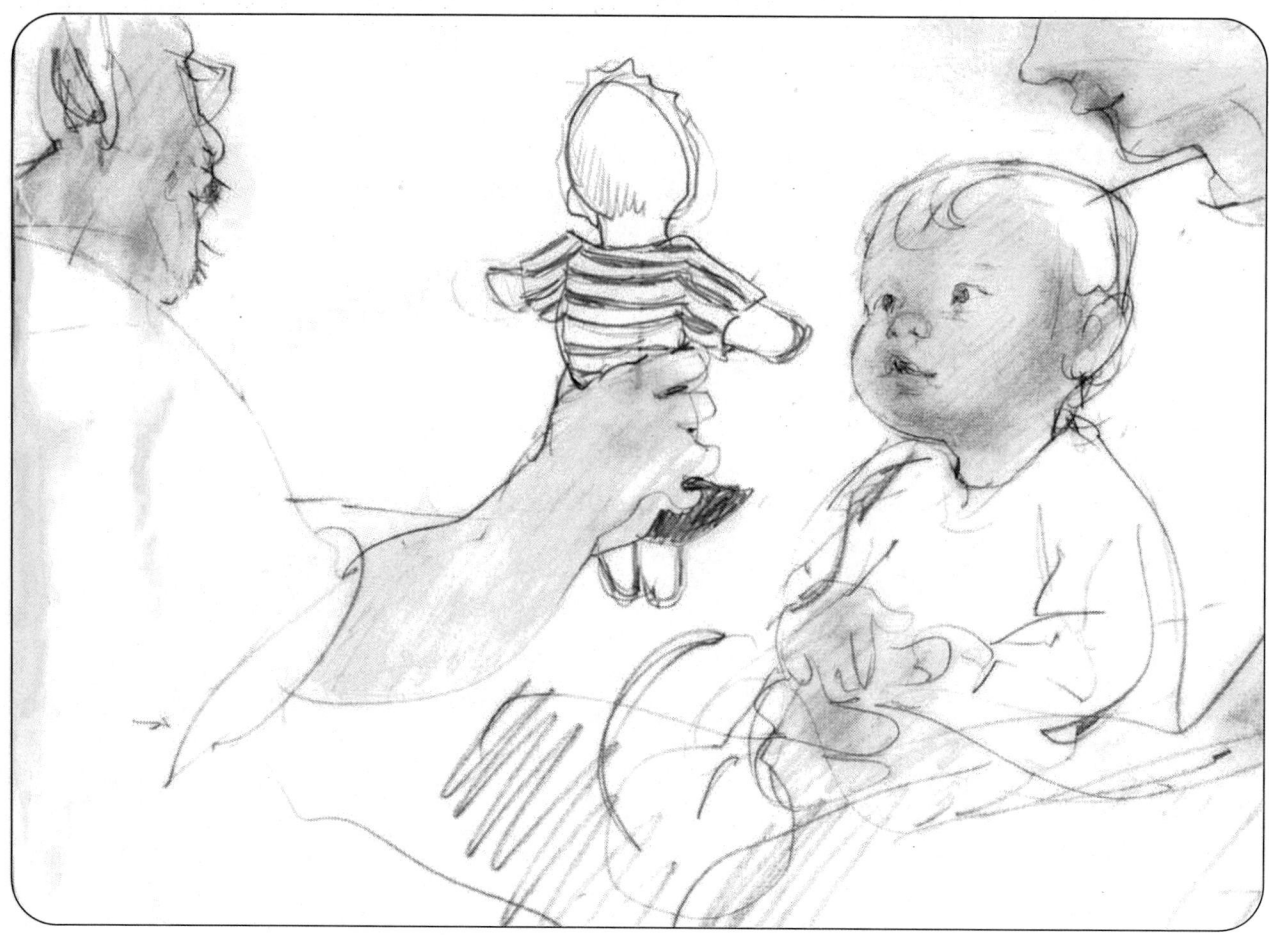

VISUAL SPHERE is the visual awareness distance, the space within which a child looks at interesting visual objects of certain size, color, contrast and speed of movement. We need to discover the child's visual sphere so we know where to present toys and ourselves. Place all objects within the child's visual field during the assessment.

VISUAL ATTENTION is the equal awareness of objects on either side of midline. This is an important area to assess for obvious reasons, but also because preferential looking techniques are used during the assessment that may require visual attention. Research indicates that infants prefer moving objects, faces and black and white objects, so utilize these approaches to stimulate vision.

EXPECTED OUTCOMES...
The child should have a visual sphere of at least three feet away and respond visually without having to pair the object with sound, movement or light.

There should not be an obvious difference in the preference between the opposite halves of the visual fields, between right and left and up and down.

PROCEDURE: Visual Sphere

1) Place the child in the best position for comfort and motor stability and head control.

2) In order to get a response or decrease visual distractions you may need to wiggle objects, move them closer or place them in front of a plain background.

3) Interact in a way that is appropriate for the particular child. If there is still no response move the object slowly in the child's periphery, alternating sides to determine if the child responds only to one side.

4) Air movement can cause a reaction not visually initiated, so take care not to cause a breeze by moving too fast.

5) Whenever there are signs the child is losing interest discontinue using that stimulus and play with something else for a while.

6) If you see the child maintains interest beyond 5 feet, use smaller targets then measure his or her visual sphere.

7) Present an interesting high contrast object close to the child and then move it away to measure the visual sphere.

8) Observe & record the distance at which the child loses interest in looking at the toy.

PROCEDURE: Visual Attention

1) Place the child in the best position for comfort and motor stability and head control.

2) To compare the functions of the right and left field halves choose pairs of interesting objects, place them in front of you.

3) By presenting objects of different sizes and interest values, and at different distances from midline, one can see which visual field half (right or left of midline) entices the child's visual fixation the most.

4) If there seems to be a strong preference for fixating on one side, one can quantify the observation further by using unequal objects, e.g., increase size difference so object on the preferred side is smaller than the object on the non-preferred side.

5) If the upper and lower fields have equal preference and there is a clear difference in preference between the horizontal field halves, use vertical presentation of targets in all test situations.

6) If the child has horizontal nystagmus, responses are easier to notice when the targets are presented vertically.

7) Where there is no preference, present targets either horizontally or vertically. Use the findings in the child's visual stimulation program and teach the child to shift attention.

BE CONCERNED IF...
- ❏ No visual responses are noted.
- ❏ The child's visual sphere is closer than 24 inches after 1 month of age.
- ❏ The child only responds if the object is paired with movement, sounds or lights.
- ❏ You do not get an equal response to the objects in each eye above, below, right and left of midline.

BE PLEASED IF...

Visual responses are noted in children who do not generally react visually, record observations.

Child's visual sphere is within 3 feet.

Child has equal visual responses in each eye.

FIXATION

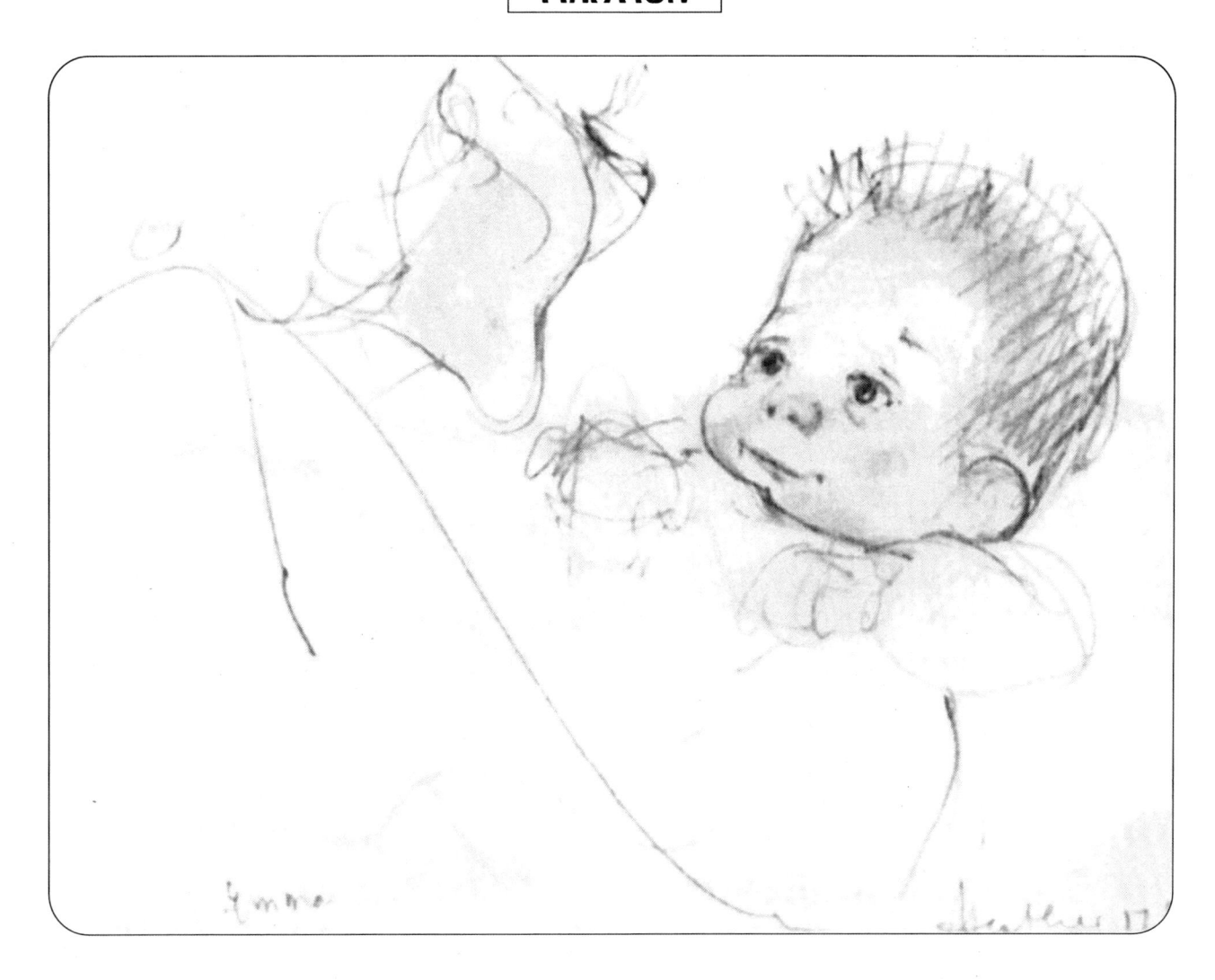

Some visually impaired children seem to look past objects when looking toward them. This may indicate, among other possibilities, that the child's central vision does not function and he or she uses eccentric fixation (retinal area other than the fovea of the macula used for visual fixation). Some children with ROP have their retina pulled by scar tissue so that the macula (area of the retina responsible for acute central vision) is more lateral than in a normal eye. The child may appear to have strabismus, an eye turn, when actually he/she is using foveal vision. (Hyvärinen L., & Appleby, K., 1996)

It is always important to describe how the child fixates. If the child has strabismus (eye misalignment), one has to find out which eye the child uses, or whether he/she constantly changes the fixating eye, which makes test situations very difficult to interpret. Look for children with rapid eye movement (nystagmus). In addition, some children may need to turn their heads or eyes in unusual positions in order to fixate on a target. This may be due to the need for eccentric fixation.

EXPECTED OUTCOMES WHEN COMPARED TO "TYPICAL" VISUAL DEVELOPMENT...
Nothing unusual about fixation is noted.

PROCEDURE:

1) Place the child in the best position for comfort and motor stability and head control.

2) Use a motivating toy or object, which may be your face, a very powerful fixation target for infants.

3) Note the toy or object at which the child fixates.

4) Observe if he or she avoids looking.

5) Observe how the child looks at the toy, i.e., head and eye position.

6) Record the distance at which he or she stops looking at the toy.

7) If the child's eyes look as if they are in an unusual position, record the position on the Recording Form from the Appendix.

BE CONCERNED IF...
- An eye looks as if it turns in or out.
- The toy has to be held very close before the child pays attention.
- The child avoids looking or does not respond visually.
- A child fixates with head tilt or turn.
- Direct eye contact is absent as if the child is fixating beyond toy.
- Lack of eye contact or fixation by 3 months.
- There is a lack of fixation or avoidance of fixation.
- Rapid eye movement is noted.

BE PLEASED IF...
Any visual responses are noted in children who do not generally react visually, note your observations.

Child fixates directly at the target.

No unusual head or eye position in noted.

MUSCLE BALANCE

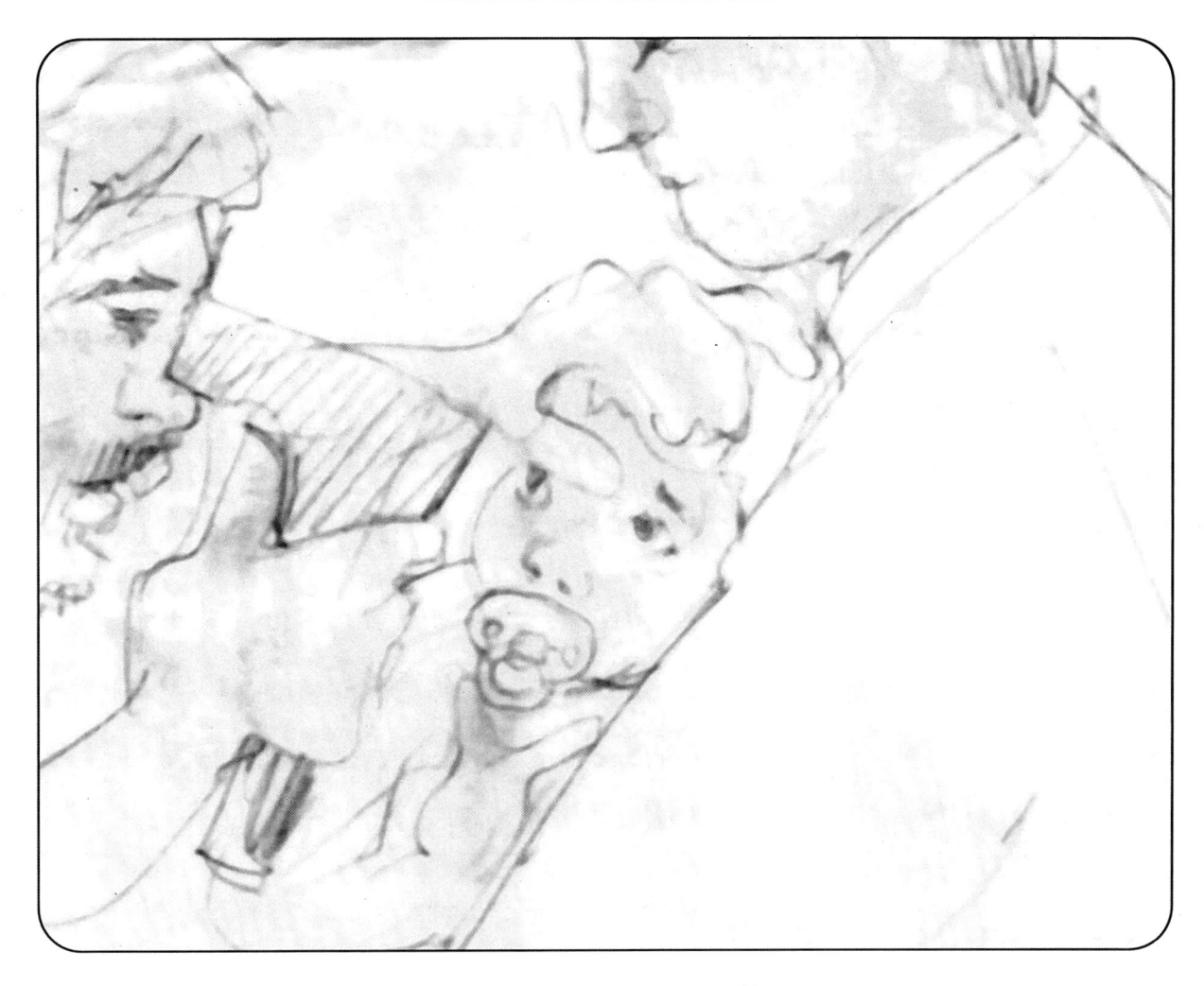

"If for any reason a child does not gain unity of full eye teaming, this deficiency can become a great deterrent to all judgements of spatial orientation, relationships, depth perception, and–more important–the immediacy and accuracy of clear, single vision for almost every object or symbol in the usual classroom program." (Optometric Extension Program, prepared by, Section on Children's Vision Care and Guidance.)

When the two eyes do not focus at precisely the same place at the same time, a child may lose his or her place when reading, reverse letters or words, or even see double. Small misalignments causing doubling can create serious reading problems in children (Richards, 1984).

Some of the terms you may encounter in doctor reports are explained below: Esotropia, Esophoria, Exotropia, Exophoria, Hypertropia, and Hyperphoria. When I report my findings I explain which eye turned in or out rather than use these terms, since I do not diagnosis and only report my observations.

Strabismus is an eye condition referred to as eye turn, misalignment, crossed eyes, deviating eye, etc. The eye turn is due to extraocular muscle imbalance and is not the same as "lazy eye" (amblyopia: suppression of an eye). The eye turn may occur while fixating (looking at) distance objects, near objects or both. When there is an eye turn both eyes do not always fixate simultaneously at the same time at the same object and affects stereo vision and binocular depth perception.

Eso

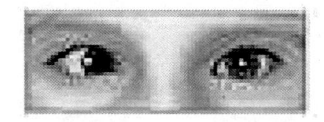

Exo

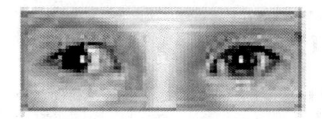

Hyper

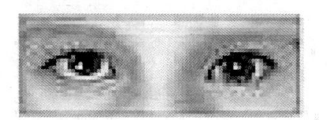

Eso refers to one eye turning "in" (toward nose) and the other eye centered. See the penlight reflection is on the outer (temporal) portion of the iris shown in the top picture below.

Exo refers to one eye turning "out" (away from nose) and the other eye centered. See the penlight reflection is on the inner (nasal) portion of the iris shown in the middle picture below.

Hyper refers to an eye turn "up" or "down". See the penlight reflection is on the "lower" portion of the iris shown in the bottom picture below when the right eye turns "up".

Tropia: When an eye turn occurs all of the time, it is called "constant strabismus" (tropia), esotropia, exotropia, hypertropia.

Phoria: When an eye turn occurs only some of the time, it is called "intermittent strabismus" (phoria). For example with intermittent strabismus, an eye turn might be observed only from time to time, such as during stressful situations or when the person is not feeling well.

It doesn't matter if the strabismus is "constant" or "intermittent", it always requires evaluation and treatment, as children do not outgrow strabismus.

http://www.strabismus.org/strabismus_crossed_eyes.html

EXPECTED OUTCOMES WHEN COMPARED TO "TYPICAL" VISUAL DEVELOPMENT...

Good visual development includes eye muscles that control the paired eyes so that they "team" and the two eyes exhibit fusion and perform as one. No eye turn should be noted in either eye when the other eye is fixating. The penlight reflection should be centered in both pupils during direct reflection. No eye movement should be noted during alternate cover and each eye should have a centered penlight reflection during cover/uncover.

PROCEDURE:
Do not use a penlight with seizure prone children

1) Place the child in the best position for comfort and motor stability and head control.

2) Hold a penlight between the child's eyes, at eye level, 18" from the nose. Briefly shine the light in the child's eyes.

3) Note the penlight's reflections on the pupils (direct reflection).

4) Mark the location of the reflections on the drawing of the eyes on the Recording Form from the appendix.

5) Place an animal cover over the penlight and hold it in front of the child's eyes, as above.

6) Place your fingers lightly on the child's head (if tolerated), or quickly place your thumb (from above) in front of the child's eye without touching the head, as you alternately cover the eyes (alternate cover).

7) Cover one eye and quickly uncover it and observe that eye to see its position as it attempts to fixate on the animal penlight cover (cover/uncover).

BE CONCERNED IF...
- The penlight reflection isn't centered simultaneously in each pupil when shining it in the eyes.
- Either eye moves as an eye is uncovered and the child tries to look at the animal on the penlight.
- Be concerned also if you observe any of the following muscle imbalances: During direct reflection either eye turns or either eye turns out while other eye is straight.
- During direct reflection either eye deviates either upward or downward while the other is straight.
- During alternate cover eye movement is noted.
- During cover/uncover the eye at rest is not aligned straight as determined by the reflection of the light on the pupil.

BE PLEASED IF...
The reflection of the penlight is centered symmetrically in each pupil during the direct reflection portion of the assessment.

No eye movement is noted during alternate cover.

The eye at rest during cover/uncover testing maintains central fixation.

VISUALLY FOLLOWING MOVING TOY/OCULAR PURSUITS

When a child has difficulty with ocular pursuits there may be a peripheral disturbance in the function of one the muscles of the eye or paralysis. More seldom it is a central disturbance causing gaze paralysis, i.e., the muscle function is present but the command function may fail. Therefore the child cannot look in a certain direction. Whenever you observe a dysfunction in this area that has not been reported, inform the child's doctor. (Hyvärinen, L. & Appleby, K. (1996))

Children who are motorically involved may also have eye muscles that are compromised and may not be able to get their eyes into all positions of gaze (motility).

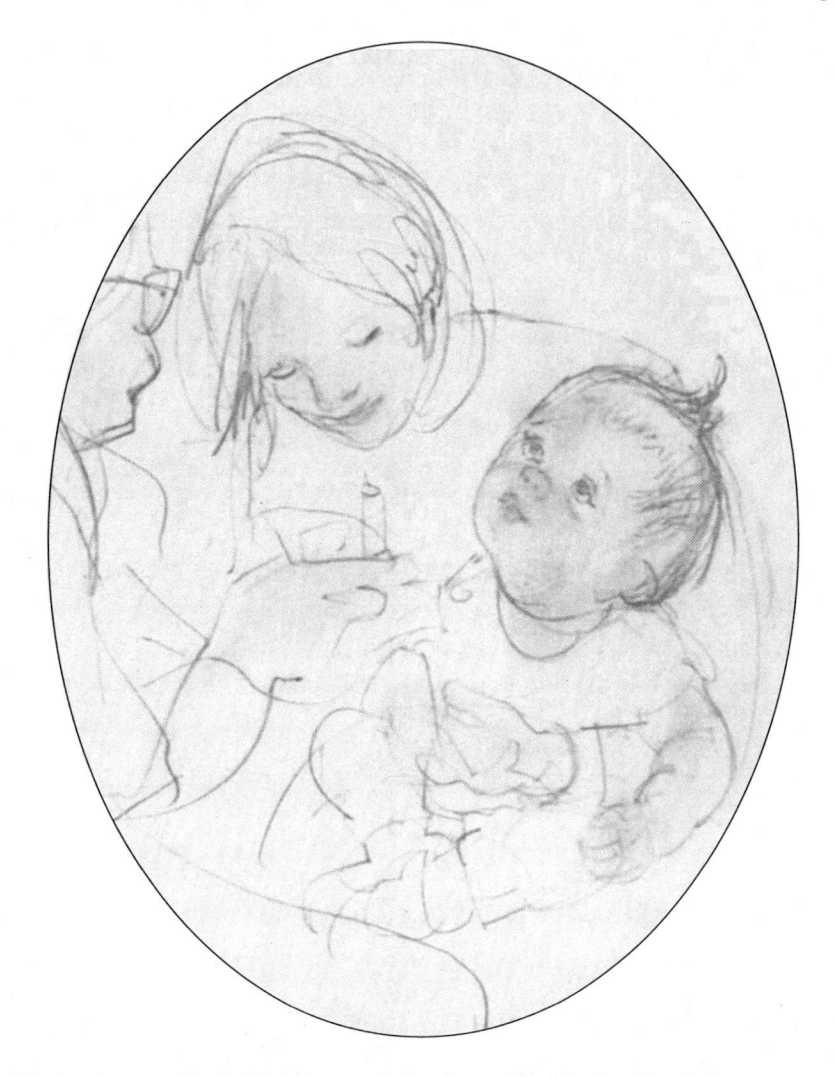

EXPECTED OUTCOMES WHEN COMPARED TO "TYPICAL" VISUAL DEVELOPMENT...
A young child should be able to visually follow a moving toy with smooth eye movements as it moves horizontally, vertically, diagonally and in a circle, without head movement.

PROCEDURE:

1) Place the child in the best position for comfort, motor stability and head control.

2) Use a motivating toy paired with sound or light if needed to attract a child's gaze.

3) Move the toy slowly horizontally and then vertically while watching the child's eyes as he or she visually follows the toy and observe head position.

4) If the child can visually follow without head movement with eye movement only, can child visually cross midline without moving head

5) If the child turns his or her head when watching the target move, rather than only moving his or her eyes, try holding his or her head, if tolerated.

6) If one eye lags in a certain direction check the function when the other eye is covered.

7) Hold the child's head still, if tolerated, and see if he or she can get into all extreme positions of gaze (motility).

BE CONCERNED IF...

- By 1 year of age child needs to use head movement, rather than eye movement alone.
- The child can not visually follow the moving toy in one or more directions by 3 months.
- The eye movement is off pace with the movement of the toy.
- Look for difficulty visually crossing midline, jerky eye movements and frequent breaks in fixation, i.e., blink or look away.
- When the head is held the child struggles to move his/her body in order to watch the moving toy.
- The child can not get his/her eyes into all extreme positions of gaze.
- One eye turns while the other lags.

BE PLEASED IF...

Any visual responses are noted in children who do not generally react visually.

If the child, by 1 year of age is able to visually follow a moving object in all direction with eye movement and no head movement.

MOVEMENT OF BOTH EYES INWARD/CONVERGENCE

Convergence is related to the ability of the brain to unite the image of an object, created in each eye, into a single image. Simultaneous inward movement of both eyes, toward each other, usually is an effort to maintain single binocular vision as object approaches. (Cassin, B., Solomon, S., Rubin, M. 1990).

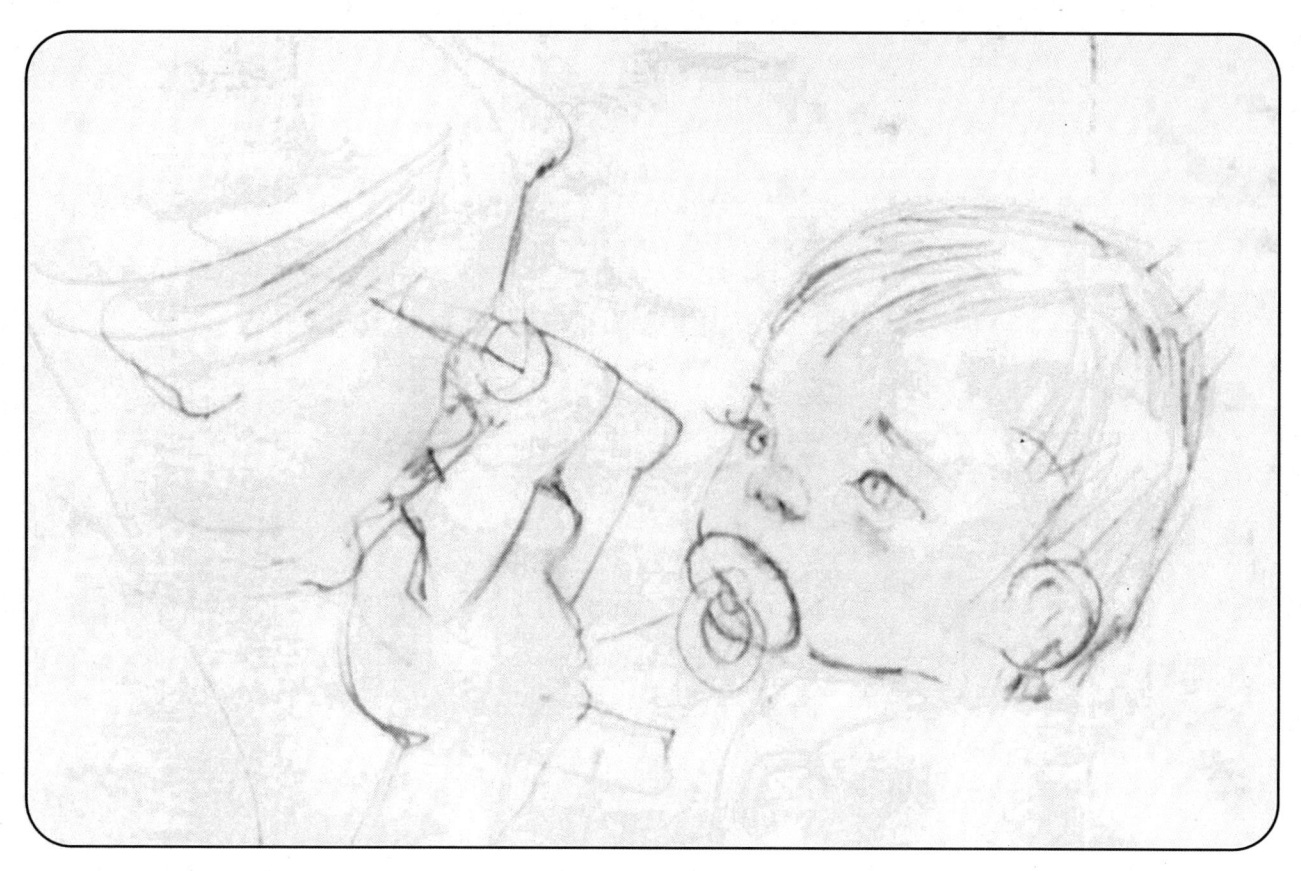

Reading requires unique eye movement skills. Initially, the eyes must turn in and rotate to converge so both eyes are pointed at or aligned on the word or words being inspected. If a child cannot converge his or her eyes in a smooth easy motion, fixation or clarity can not be maintained when trying to read. If a child suffers from severe convergence insufficiency, he may have intermittent double vision at near point which promotes visual stress (Richards, 1984).

Children who have difficulties converging their eyes or maintaining stable convergence often times have difficulty with academic near task such as reading and handwriting.

EXPECTED OUTCOMES WHEN COMPARED TO "TYPICAL" VISUAL DEVELOPMENT...

By 6 months of age convergence can be noted in a baby. By one year of age a child should be able to maintain fixation on the target as it moves toward his/her nose to about 3". The eyes should turn in equally and smoothly as toy moves closer.

PROCEDURE...

1) Place the child in the best position for comfort and motor stability and head control.

2) Hold whatever the child is motivated to look at, centered at eye level 18" from his or her nose and move it slowly toward the nose.

3) Note the distance the child's eyes stop turning in equally and smoothly as the toy gets closer and at what distance he or she stops fixating.

BE CONCERNED IF...
- ❑ The child's eyes stop turning in equally and smoothly
- ❑ If he/she stops fixating at the toy when it is more than 3" from his or her nose, if older than 6 months.
- ❑ If one eye turns out as the toy gets closer.
- ❑ If the eyes appear to wiggle slightly, as if not being able to maintain tight fixation.

BE PLEASED IF...
Visual responses are noted in children who do not generally react visually.

The child's eyes turn in equally and smoothly and steady fixation is maintained up to 3-4 inches.

SHIFT OF GAZE/SACCADES

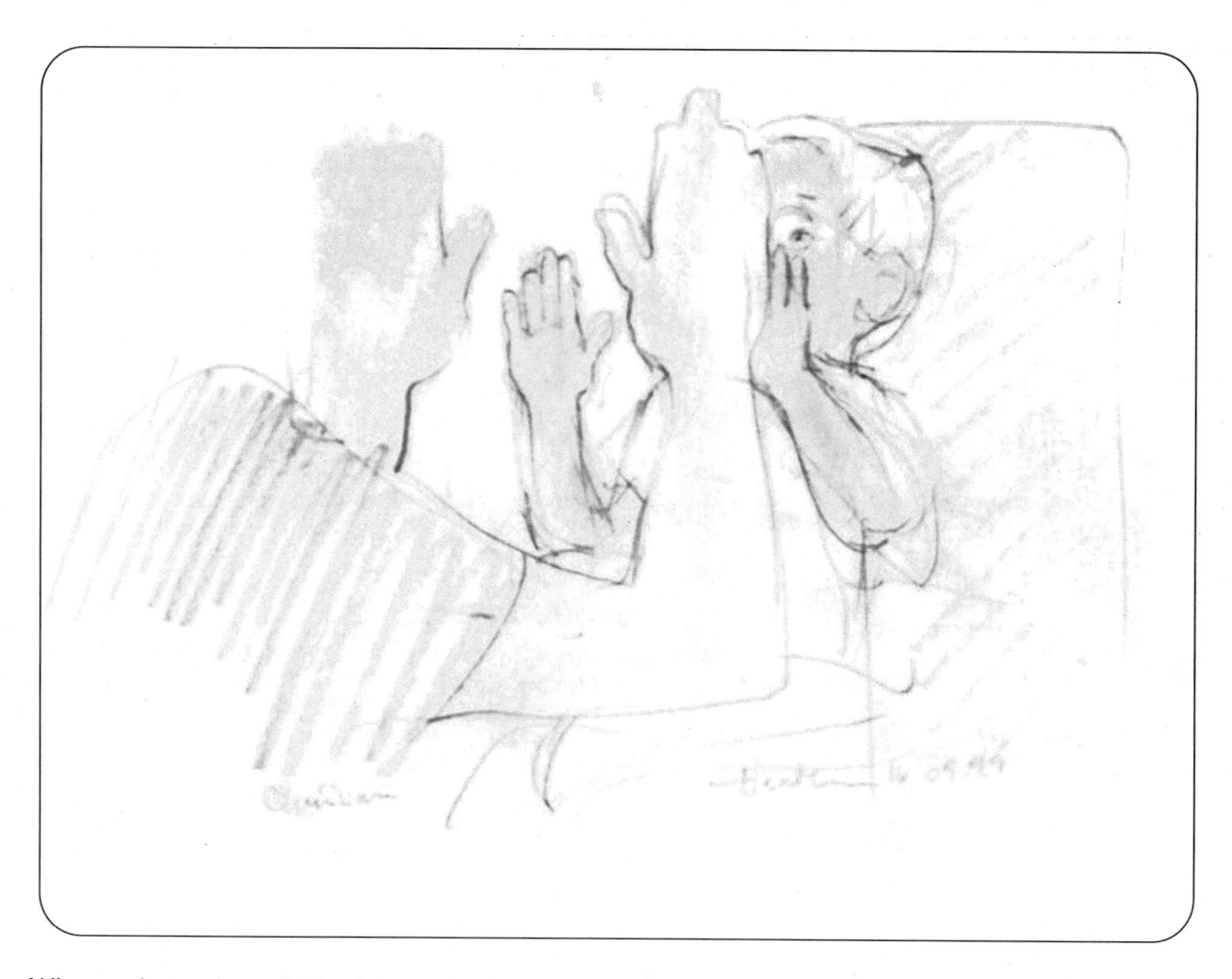

When observing shift of gaze between two fixations, pay attention to how the child re-fixates gaze on each side of midline. Also observe if fixation is broken crossing midline. This applies to both horizontal and vertical presentation. The ability to perform saccades (shift of gaze) is a prerequisite in many test situations. For example, when measuring grating acuities the child needs to shift gaze horizontally across midline to the grating paddles held on either side of midline. If the child can not do this you may need to reposition the paddles to a vertical placement,

EXPECTED OUTCOMES WHEN COMPARED TO "TYPICAL" VISUAL DEVELOPMENT...
The ability to complete saccades across midline normally appears at about 3 months of age. Before then the child may use simple saccades, several eye movements or a combination of eye and head movement to fixate from midline to more peripheral targets and/or to cross midline. The younger the child, or the further away from midline the objects are, the more likely there will be combined eye and head movement. The child should be able to smoothly shift gaze from target to target across midline, horizontally and vertically with eye movement only.

PROCEDURE:

1) Place the child in the best position for comfort and motor stability and head control.

2) Encourage the child to look directly ahead by interesting him/her in your face by singing, clicking your tongue, wearing a red clown's nose, or whatever it takes.

3) Observe how the child performs a saccade from midline to a target, then horizontally across midline by using two motivating objects, equal distance from midline.

4) Repeat with the targets presented vertically above and below midline.

5) Use your face as the midline target and get the child to fixate on it. Wiggle or squeak the object on either side of midline at the level of the child's face. Repeat with the stimulus on the other side.

6) When the child fixates on the object, wiggle or squeak another interesting object to initiate a shift of fixation.

7) If the child responds, decrease the use of the sound stimulus and use motion only to eliminate sound localization.

8) Use different distances between the two objects to determine the angle at which the child starts using combined head and eye movement.

9) If the child uses head movement to shift gaze across midline, ask another person to gently touch the child's head to reduce head movement.

10) Determine if this assists the child to move his/her eyes without head movement in order to perform proper saccades.

11) Use large objects initially when training the child to differentiate eye movements from head movements and progress to using smaller objects when the child masters the correct movement with large objects.

12) Encourage the child to look straight ahead before you present the 2 toys. If using lighted toys you may have to dim the room lights.

13) Use two matching toys with sound and/or light and hold one in each hand, at child's eye level. Place a toy in line with each eye on either side of midline equal distance apart.

14) Alternately light each toy to encourage the child to shift gaze from right to left and from left to right of midline.

15) Reposition the toys above and below midline and alternately light each toy to see if the child can shift gaze from top to bottom and from bottom to top of midline.

BE CONCERNED IF...
❑ The child can not smoothly shift gaze when looking from one toy to another. For example, the child's eyes may make several jerky movements before fixation on the second toy.
❑ The child can not shift gaze across midline without breaking fixation or blinking.
❑ The child needs to use head movement to shift gaze.

BE PLEASED IF...
Any visual responses are noted in children who do not generally react visually.

The child can smoothly shift gaze across midline and in all directions presented.

VISUAL FIELD PERIPHERAL RESPONSE TO TOYS

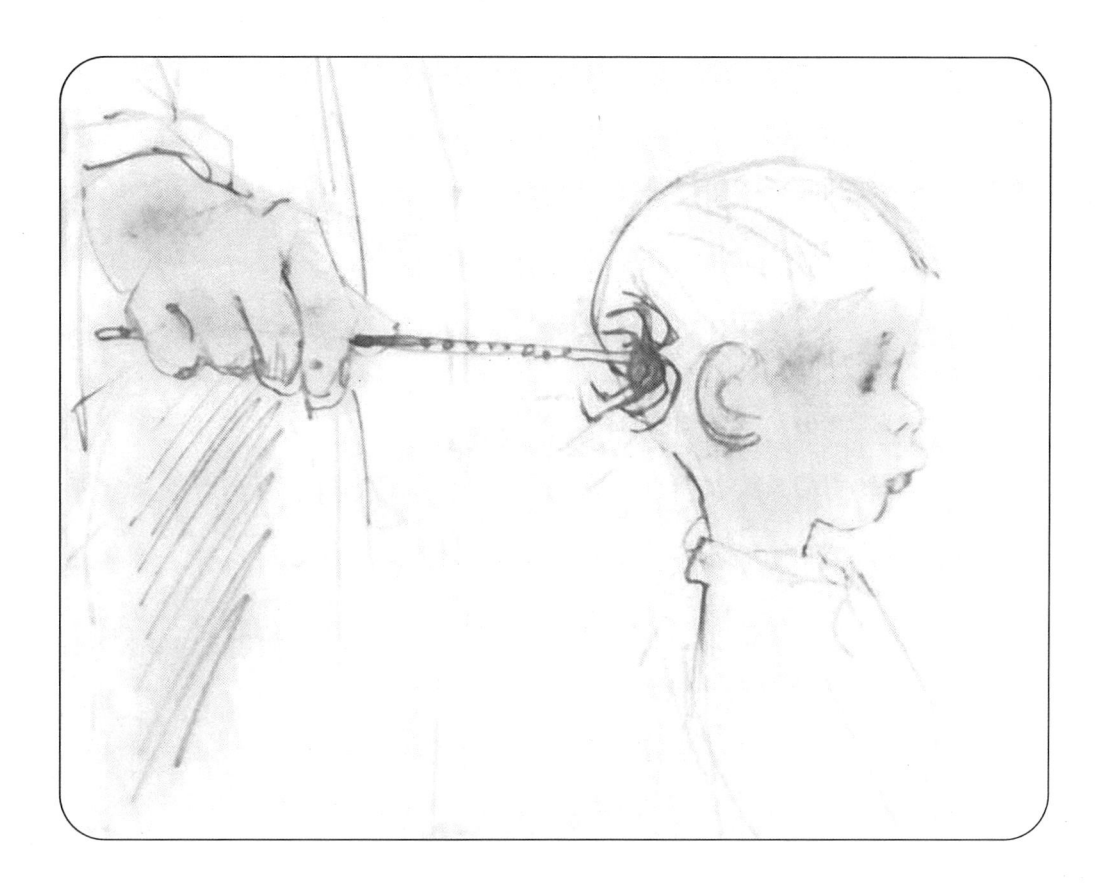

Visual Field/Field of Vision is the extent of space visible to an eye as it fixates straight ahead. In formal assessment it is measured in degrees away from fixation. (Cassin, B., Solomon, S., Rubin, M. 1990). In functional vision assessment the field of vision can be approximately measured by using interesting objects in order to determine the extremes of a child's visual field. Large objects can easily be detected in a functioning peripheral visual field. Central visual field is difficult to assess in infants and in children with multihandicaps.

EXPECTED OUTCOMES WHEN COMPARED TO "TYPICAL" VISUAL DEVELOPMENT...
By one year old a child's visual development should include upper visual fields reaching adult size while horizontal and lower fields that are smaller than adult size (Mohn & Hof-van-Duin, 1986).

PROCEDURE:

1) Place the child in the best position for comfort and motor stability and head control.

2) Utilize the following steps with difficult to test children.

3) Have a helper stand behind the child.

4) The tester, in front of the child, tries to get the child to fixate on his or her face and signals the helper when fixation is straightforward.

5) The helper then moves a motivating object forward from behind the child, about 10" from child's head.

6) In a test situation like this, the child has two competing targets for his/her attention, the face of the tester and the object that appears from the periphery. The tester's face is such an emotionally strong target that it may effectively prevent a shift of fixation to the object.

7) It is possible to decrease the effect of the tester's face by getting behind a poster board with a peek hole in the center.

8) Talk to the child while peeking above the poster board to bring the child's gaze to midline.

9) Move behind the poster board and look through the peek hole as the helper presents the object peripherally.

10) Repeat by presenting the target several times coming from the left, right, above and below midline.

11) Note at which point in the field of vision the child notices the object and place an "X" on the Recording Form found in the Appendix.

12) Compare these results with your observations at free play when balls or other playthings appear from behind the child.

13) Record observations on the Recording Form found in the Appendix.

BE CONCERNED IF...
❑ The child has a delay turning to look at the toy as it moves into range.
❑ If you do not get an equal response to the objects in each eye above, below, right and left of midline.

BE PLEASED IF...
Any visual responses noted in children who do not generally react visually.
6-mo & older should turn to the target at the first marking on drawing on the Recording Form.

ACUITY

TYPES OF ACUITY

There are several types of acuity that are measured based on a child's ability and levels of development. Select the presentation most appropriate for each child.

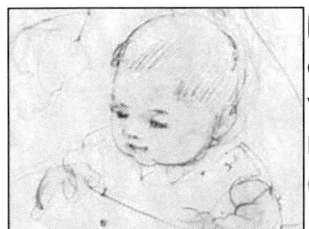

Functional (detection) Acuity: Ability to see whether or not an object, e.g., a circular target, is present in an otherwise empty visual field. Forms the basis of perimetric tests. Acuity is determined from the minimum size, which permits visibility. (Thompson, C., 1993)

Example: Detection acuity is demonstrated when a child is observed looking toward a functional object like a toy, etc. You can obtain a "functional acuity" by determining the smallest object at the greatest distance the child maintains visual contact with the object. This does not represent the most comfortable viewing distance. Place objects closer for daily tasks.

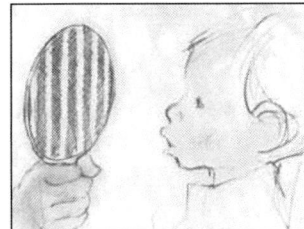

Grating (resolution) Acuity: Ability to discriminate two or more spatially separated targets. The stimulus is often a black and white striped grating, which appears gray if not resolved. Acuity is recorded as the minimum separation, which permits discrimination. (Thompson, C., 1993)

Example: Resolution acuity includes grating acuity measured in cycles per degree.

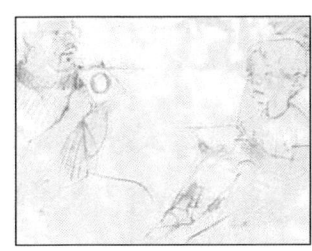

Optotype (recognition) Acuity: The measure of the eye's ability to distinguish object details and shape (symbol, number, letter). Assessed by the smallest identifiable object {optotype} that can be seen at a specified distance, usually 20 feet for distance and 16 inches for near. (Cassin, B., Solomon, S., Rubin, M. 1990)

Example: Typical eye charts for young children include symbols, which is an example of optotype measurement. Optotype measurement is preferred for the most accurate measurement of acuity. However, not all children are able to respond to this level of assessment.

Early correction of vision in young children is extremely important. If an infant has accommodation difficulties or is hyperopic/farsighted (see better at distance than at near) and visual communication is disturbed, proper near correction lenses must be prescribed as soon as the difficulty in interaction becomes diagnosed, usually at the age of 3-4 months. If hyperopia is high, 6 diopters or more, glasses need to be prescribed even earlier. A practical difficulty at that age is to find good frames that fit such little faces (Hyvärinen, 2000).

FUNCTIONAL (detection) ACUITY

EXPECTED OUTCOMES WHEN COMPARED TO "TYPICAL" VISUAL DEVELOPMENT...
The child will be able to look at tiny objects at near and small objects at distance as an example of **functional acuity**.

PROCEDURE...
1) Place the child in best position for comfort, motor stability & head control.

2) If possible try to cover an eye so you can evaluate each eye.

3) Be sure the child stopped participating due to the task and not because he/she has lost interest. For example use soccer balls decreasing in size from about 5" to 1 inch, or toys that are identical, decreasing in size appropriate to the child's responsiveness

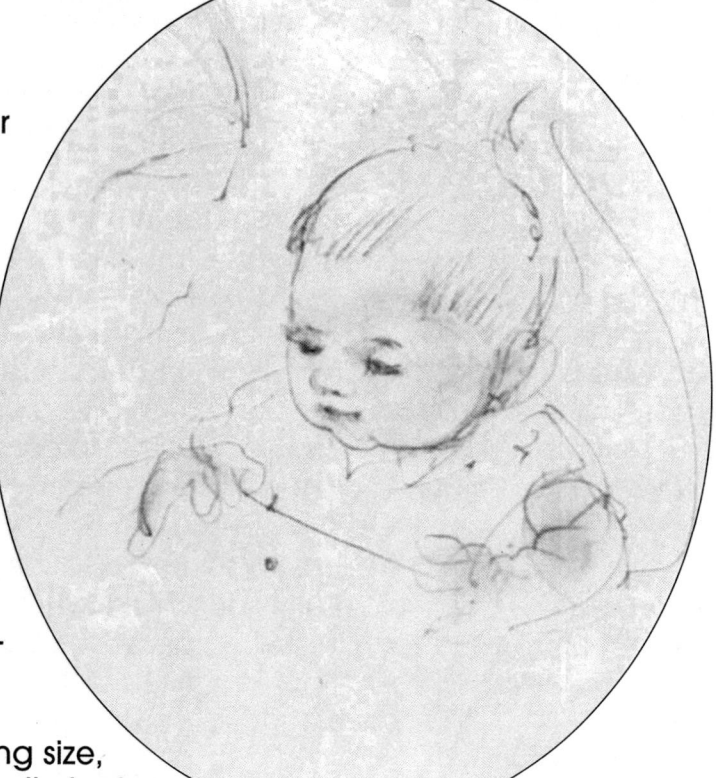

4) Use identical objects of decreasing size, if possible, e.g., soccer balls. This eliminates the possibility of the child looking at the object that is most interesting and not in relationship to the size of the object.

5) Determine and record the smallest toy responded to and the furthest distance away from the child it was before he/she stopped looking.

6) Use a larger target if the toy is too small. and position further back.

7) Record the smallest size toy and the furthest distance it was from the child before he/she stopped looking.

8) Do both eyes and each eye individually, if possible.

9) Some children may tolerate wearing "one eyed sunglasses" to occlude an eye.

BE CONCERNED IF...
☐ The child does not look at the toys or needs to be closer than 3" away to see it.
☐ If the child only responds to large toys.

BE PLEASED IF...
Any visual responses are noted in children who do not generally react visually.
The child responds to all the toys presented within his/her visual sphere.

GRATING (resolution) ACUITY

A child's response or lack of response to certain size grating patterns is not solely a measure of his or her resolution ability. The child's response is also dependent on his or her interest in the objects, attention span, physical needs, etc. This is why it is necessary to observe the child before the assessment to determine normal behaviors to certain conditions. A play situation offers an environment that encourages natural responses which maximizes the child's performance.

Preferential looking (PL) situations require that the child either makes a saccade (shift of gaze) without head movement from midline to the object, or turns his/her head from midline to fixate on the object. Present objects vertically if the child has horizontal nystagmus (rapid eye movement) or difficulty with horizontal movements and not with vertical movements. If the only response is some sign of awareness such as a smile, you can still try to determine whether there is a difference between the child's reaction when the gray paddle is presented simultaneously with a grating paddle.

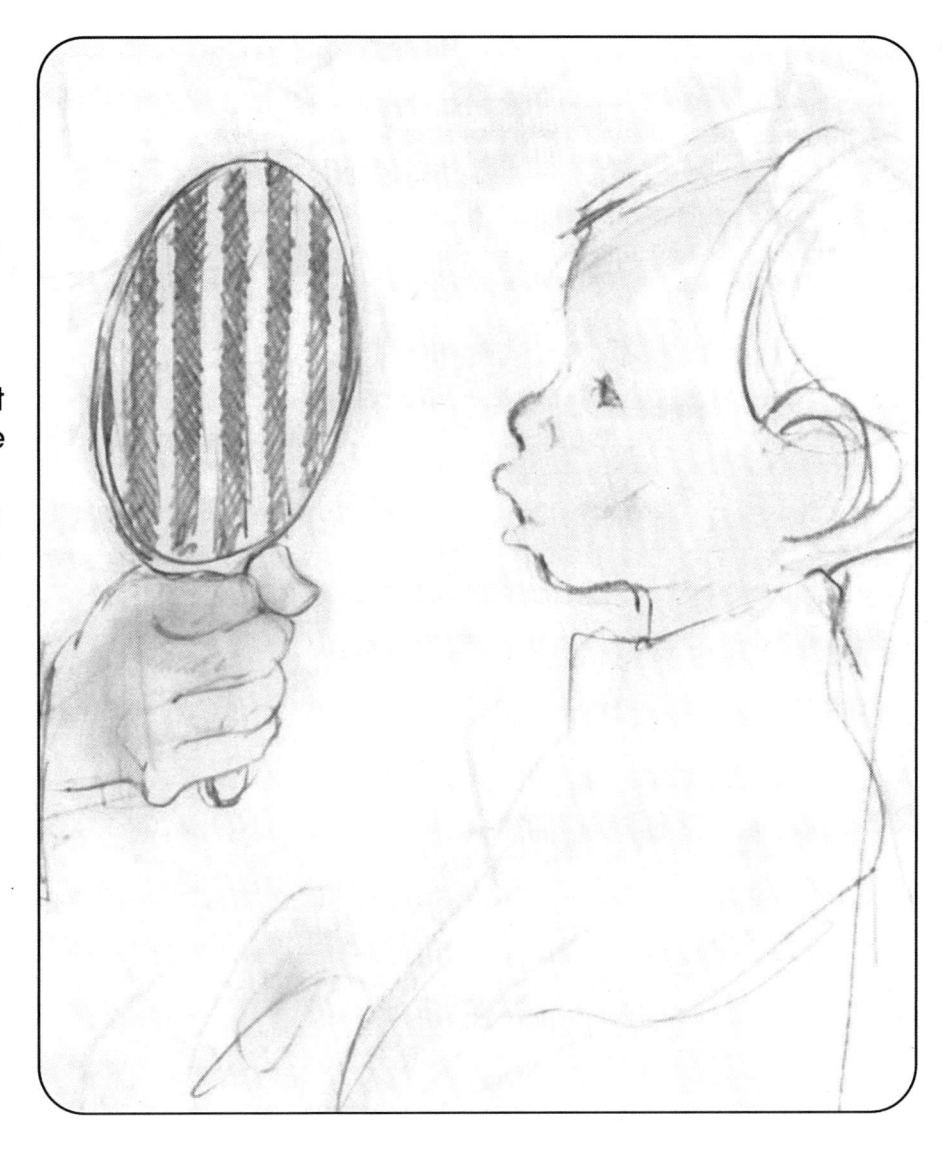

Some children with a very poor peripheral visual system cannot see even broad black and white stripes at high contrast. Frequently the reason a child does not react is due to the loss of visual attention, (attentional deficit). It is important to assess a child's visual sphere & visual attention, fixation, ocular pursuits, saccades, visual field, in that order, before assessing approximate grating acuities. This will assist in eliminating errors in interpreting the child's responses to PL techniques.

WHAT ARE GRATINGS AND CYCLE PER DEGREE

One cpd means: one cycle equals one dark and one white stripe within one degree of angle of vision. One degree of visual angle equates to 1 centimeter (cm) at a distance of 57 cm (22.5"). For example, picture 180 degrees by spreading both arms straight out from your sides. Look straight ahead and visualize one degree. It would be like a slice of pie with the narrowest portion at the bridge of your nose progressing wider the further out you go. The width of the slice of pie will be exactly one centimeter wide at 22.5 " from the narrow end near your face. That is the width of the space within which one cycle (one dark and one white stripe) will fit. Thus, one centimeter equals one degree of visual angle at 22.5". The narrower the stripes on a LEA Grating paddle the more cycles will fit within the one degree of angle of vision. For example, if you have "normal" adult vision you would have a measurement of about 30cpd. The larger the number of cpd the sharper the person's vision.

On each LEA Grating paddle the frequency of the printed grating is given as cycles per centimeter (cpcm), of the surface. Thus, at 22.5 inches and only at that distance the cycles per degree value of each grating is equal to the cpcm printed on the paddle. For example, at 22.5." the 0.25 cpcm paddle is equal to 0.25 cpd. When the paddle is brought closer the number of cycles per degree decreases. When used at a distance greater than about 22.5" the number of cycles increases.

HOW TO DEVELOP PREFERENTIAL LOOKING (PL) TECHNIQUES IN CHILDREN

Introduce the child to the LEA Gratings (paddles) including the gray paddle while wearing the gray cobbler apron (available from Vision Associates). Encourage the child to look toward his/her midline by placing an interesting toy in the center of the apron. Then simultaneously place the toy and gray paddle, one on each side of the child's midline, in front of the apron at his/her eye level. Repeat after switching the positions of the toy and gray paddle. Watch to see which side the child fixates at first. Now you and the child are prepared for PL test situation.

HOW TO REPORT GRATING ACUITY IN CYCLES PER DEGREE

Information gained from gratings is useful as a means to monitor visual performance and stimulate vision in visually impaired infants and children. When LEA Gratings are used grating acuities can be obtained and reported in cycles per degree (cpd).

GRATING ACUITY VALUES SHOULD BE EXPRESSED IN CYCLES PER DEGREE (CPD) RATHER THAN IN SNELLEN NOTATION BECAUSE:

Grating acuity values are related to detection of long thin lines whereas Snellen acuities (i.e., 20/20, etc.) are related to recognition of forms. Gratings stimulate a large portion of the retina, and optotypes fire a response on the fovea (central pit in the macula that produces sharpest vision; contains a high concentration of cones...) (Cassin, B., Solomon, S., Rubin, M. 1990)

These two ways of measuring vision are related only in normal foveal vision. For example, if a child has some spotty visual field loss such as with a scotoma he or she may still respond within the levels for his age on the gratings. Thus a child may not be identified as having a vision deficit. Differences measured between grating acuity and Snellen acuity is, in some cases, 4-20 times.

At first it may be confusing getting used to the acuity expression of cycles per degree (cpd). However, it is important to use cpd and show parents how cpd values are related to the width of the lines. Thus, parents and educators can better understand the level of grating information the child is able to see at high contrast.

EXPECTED OUTCOMES WHEN COMPARED TO "TYPICAL" VISUAL DEVELOPMENT...

<u>Grating acuity</u> expected outcomes depend on the age of the child. At birth a normally sighted infant has the resolution capability of about 1 cpd and it increases to a range of 10-20 cpd in a few months. By 18 months the narrowest grating the baby responds to is between 4cpd-16cpd.

PROCEDURE:
<u>Grating Acuity:</u> Can be used with infants up to 18 months of age and/or multi-handicapped people who can not respond to optotype tests. Testing is based on preferential looking.

1) Use **LEA Gratings** and start testing at 2 feet if this distance is well within the child's visual sphere and he/she can shift gaze horizontally across midline.

2) Hold the gray paddle against a gray apron and put the largest grating (0.25 cpcm) behind the gray paddle and place them about 22" from the child, with equal movement pull each paddle out to either side of midline in opposite directions with equal speed.

3) Observe the child's eyes to see if he/or she fixates on the grating paddle rather than on the gray paddle.

4) Repeat this procedure after switching the positions of the grating and gray paddles.

5) When the child stops responding to the gratings it is most likely because he/she can no longer detect the presence of the parallel lines as they blur to gray. Be sure to determine if the child stopped looking because he/she lost interest. Repeat.

6) Note the narrowest gratings the child looked at before he/she stops fixating at 22". If the child does not respond at this distance, move closer.

7) Record the frequency of the grating (found on the paddle) on the recording form.

8) Results of these steps will indicate what the child's resolution ability is at functional distances.

9) Use the following chart to determine approximate grating acuities reported in cycles per degree (cpd).

10) Use the Graph to compare the child's performance to "typical" development.

GRATING ACUITY REPORTED IN CYCLES PER DEGREE (CPD) BASED ON THE LEA GRATINGS (PADDLES)

DISTANCE IN INCHES & CM
CYCLES PER CENTIMETER (cpcm): PRINTED ON PADDLES

GRATING ACUITY REPORTED IN CYCLES PER DEGREE (cpd)
BASED ON THE LEA GRATINGS (PADDLES)

DISTANCE IN INCHES/CM	CYCLES PER CENTIMETER (cpcm): PRINTED ON PADDLES					
	0.25	0.5	1.0	2.0	4.0	8.0
11.5"(29cm)	0.12cpd	0.25cpd	0.50cpd	1.0cpd	2.0cpd	4.0cpd
22.5"(57cm)	0.25cpd	0.50cpd	1.0cpd	2.0cpd	4.0cpd	8.0cpd
34"(86cm)	0.40cpd	0.75cpd	1.5cpd	3.0cpd	6.0cpd	12.0cpd
45"(114cm)	0.50cpd	1.0cpd	2.0cpd	4.0cpd	8.0cpd	16.0cpd
56"(142cm)	0.62cpd	1.25cpd	2.5cpd	5.0cpd	10.0cpd	20.0cpd

BE CONCERNED IF...
The child does not fall within the shaded area on the graph below.

BE PLEASED IF...
Any visual responses are noted in children who do not generally react visually.
The child responds appropriately for his/her age.

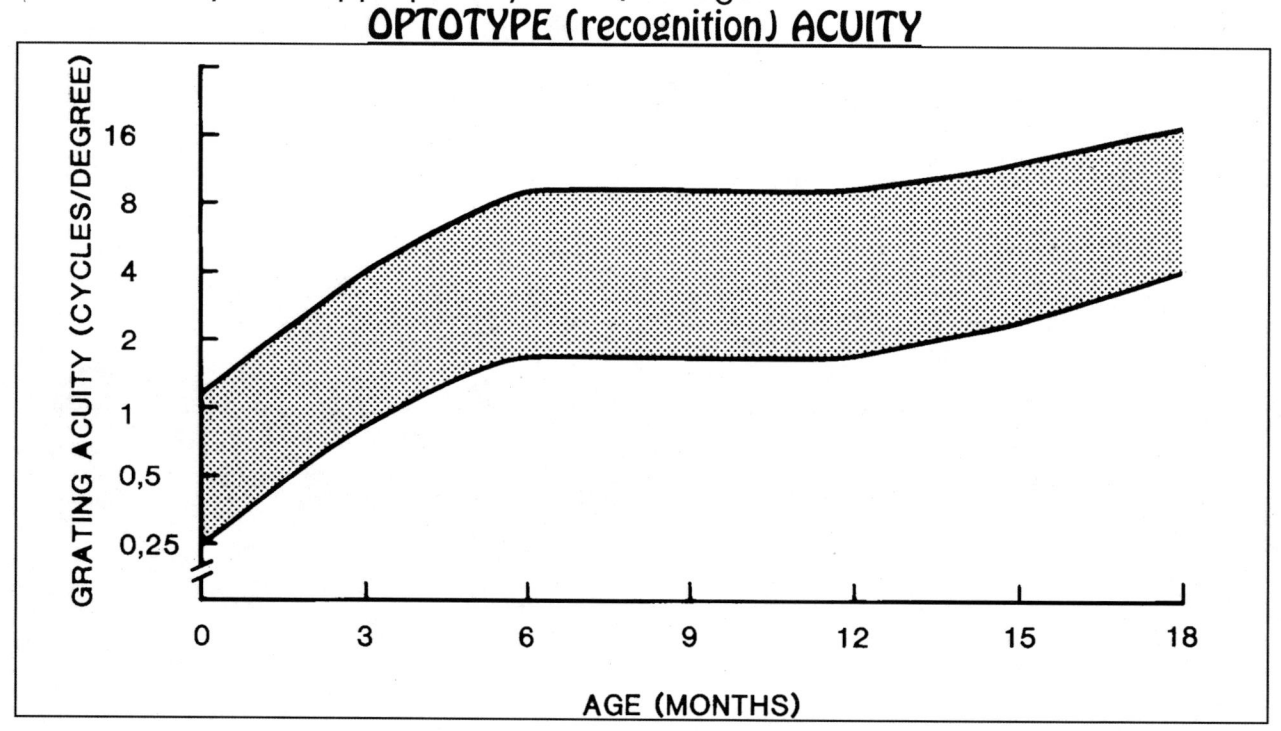

OPTOTYPE (recognition) ACUITY

EXPECTED OUTCOMES WHEN COMPARED TO "TYPICAL" VISUAL DEVELOPMENT...

When using optotype (symbols, numbers, letters) tests, recognition acuity is based on the child's age and varies from age 3 (20/40), age 5 (20/30) and age 7 (20/20).

PROCEDURE:

1) Use the following procedures if optotype testing is appropriate for the child and follow the directions included with the tests/book.

2) <u>Optotype Acuity:</u> See if the child can show you he can match the LEA symbols and identify them either by name, by pointing or by using eye gaze to the matching one.

3) <u>Near acuity:</u> Have the child identify the symbols on the **LEA Symbol Playing Cards** or in the **PÄIVI Book.**

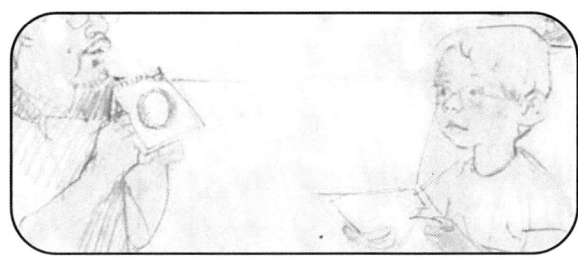

4) <u>Distance Acuity:</u> Use the **LEA Symbol FlashCards.** Record the results on the Recording Form found in the Appendix.

ADJUST TESTING DISTANCE TO SNELLEN EQUIVALENCY

Use this formula to determine Snellen equivalency when the actual test distance is different than the requirements of the chart. For example: 10 foot chart used, testing distance 5 feet and the last line of optotypes responded to and printed on the chart was 10/40.

$$\frac{\text{Viewing Distance Used}}{10 \text{ feet}} \times \text{VA value for 10 feet} = \text{Visual Acuity (VA)}$$

$$\frac{5}{10} \times \frac{10}{40} = \frac{1}{2} \times \frac{10}{40} = \frac{10}{80} = \frac{20}{160}$$

BE CONCERNED IF...

❏ The child could not identify 3 out of 5 (1 M size symbols) at near.
❏ The child could not identify 3 out of 5 (20/40 symbols) at 10'.
❏ There is a difference between responses in each eye.

BE PLEASED IF...

Child responses match the "typically" developing children section above.

CONTRAST SENSITIVITY

From my experiences, contrast sensitivity is an area in which many people have an interest in gaining further information. As I look into the research I understand exact contrast sensitivity measurements of "typically" developing infants is still being established and varies depending on the condition of measurement and the type of tests used. Some of the tests include: a variety of sine wave gratings including electronically presented, square wave gratings, low contrast optotype acuity charts, and forced choice preferential looking at decreasing contrast levels.

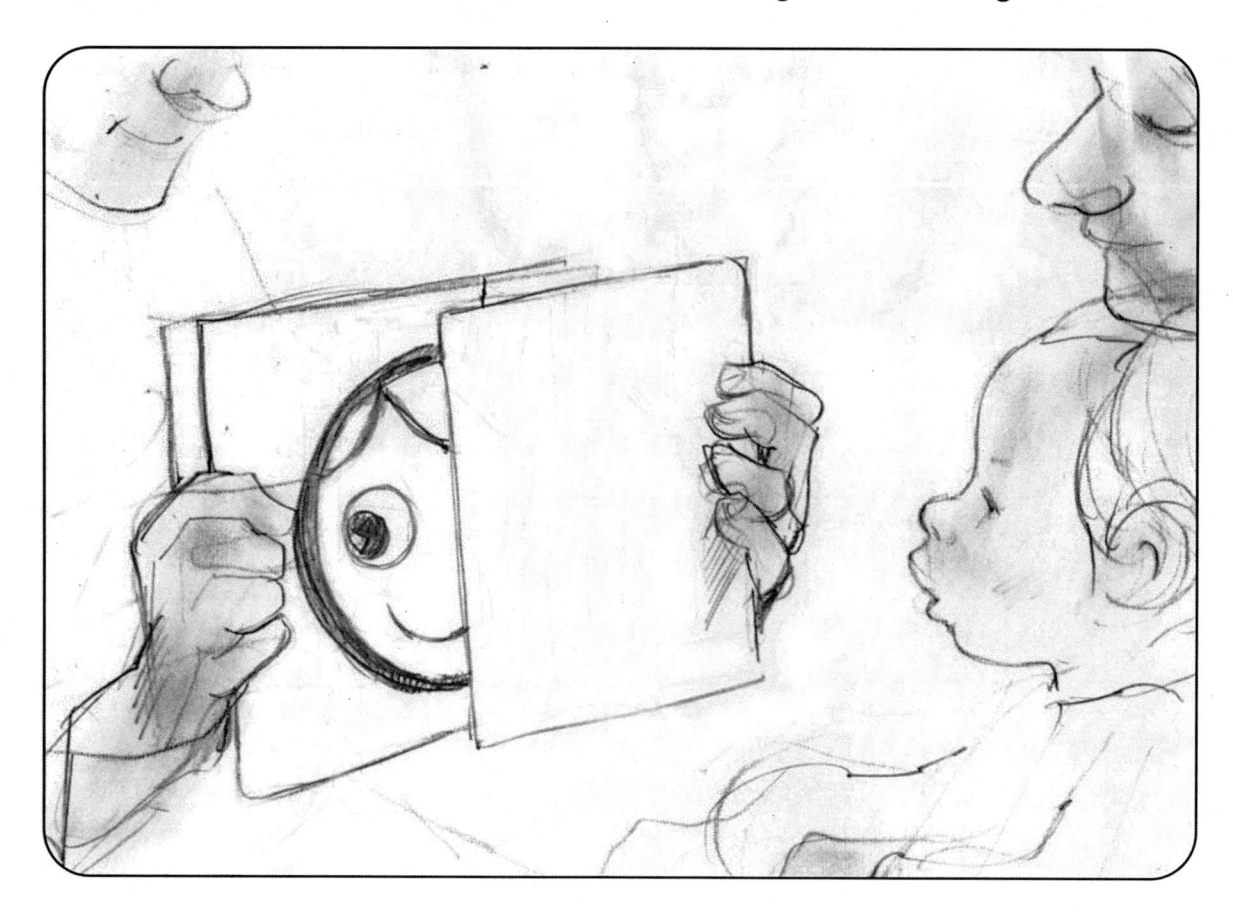

The following quotes offer some insights into contrast levels of infants. Thompson (1993) reported, "Newborns and 1 month olds do not show low-frequency attenuation and their overall sensitivity is greatly reduced. The CSF (contrast sensitivity frequency) shape is similar to that of adults, from 2 to 3 months, although shifted to lower spatial frequencies and sensitivities, particularly when obtained via behavioural means."

It appears that there are two phases in the development of contrast sensitivity (and acuity), with improvement occurring at all frequencies until 9 weeks, and only at higher spatial frequencies thereafter (Nocia, Tyler and Hamer, 1990).

An adult-like function is attained by 6-10 months using VEPs, but behavioural methods, including those of a subjective nature, suggest sensitivities are similar to adults' by about 3 years. Subsequent gradual improvement may be noted during the following few years, no doubt due as much to non-visual as neural factors (Bradley and Freeman, 1982).

WHY ASSESSMENT OF CONTRAST SENSITIVITY IS IMPORTANT...

The ability to detect objects of low contrast is an important component of the visual system. Determining the level of sensitivity offers important information for intervention and provides a base line to evaluate future changes in the development of vision. Problems with contrast sensitivity may indicate disorders that leave high contrast acuity unaffected. With some progressive eye diseases contrast sensitivity will be affected before high contrast. Thus, contrast sensitivity is an important part of visual assessment.

Visual communication is the primary mode of communicating during the first year of life. Faint shadows and changes of the contours of the mouth and eyes mediate expressions on faces require good contrast sensitivity. It is an important area to assess in infants. The "Hiding Heidi" low contrast faces accomplish this task.

Six identical "Heidi" Faces are printed in the contrast levels of: 100%, 25%, 10%, 5%, 2.5% and 1.25%. Each face is presented individually in diminishing levels of contrast until the child no longer responds. This is repeated for both eyes and each eye individually. The results indicate the lowest contrast level and furthest distance away the child responds to the face in a variety of lighting conditions.

The information gained will tell you what lighting needs are necessary for the child to respond to the six contrast levels. In order to use this information functionally, look in the mirror with the mother and compare her face with the contrast levels of "Heidi" and determine which contrast level is the closest match to her face. If the infant did not respond to the matching contrast level "Heidi" Face the mother may need to wear bright lipstick and eye liner to encourage eye contact with the infant. Eye contact between a parent and infant is a powerful stimulus to bonding. Thus, if eye contact is not present it is important for the parents to learn to facilitate eye contact and, when it is not possible, learn to use alternative ways to bond with their infant.

EXPECTED OUTCOMES WHEN COMPARED TO "TYPICAL" VISUAL DEVELOPMENT...

By 2 mos. of age the baby should be able to fixate on a person's eyes when held. By 3 months the baby should minimally respond to the 2.5% contrast level of Hiding Heidi's Face.

PROCEDURE:

1) Place child in the best position for comfort and motor stability and head control.

2) When positioning the "Hiding Heidi" Test cards, take into consideration the child's: visual sphere, fixation adaptations, shift of gaze and acuity limitations.

3) Get within the child's visual sphere, which may mean leaning over the child who is lying on the floor.

4) Try placing the "Hiding Heidi" cards about 18" from the child's face if he or she responds visually at this distance.

5) If the child can shift gaze horizontally use that movement with the "Hiding Heidi" Test. If only vertical shift of gaze is possible move the test cards vertically.

6) Turn over the card printed with "Hiding Heidi" so the blank side faces the child.

7) Place the 100% contrast "Heidi" face behind the blank card.

8) Move both cards simultaneously outward from midline and watch the child's eyes to see if the gaze goes to the "Heidi" Face. Take into consideration the child's fixation viewing position.

9) Reverse and present the "Heidi" Face on the other side. Repeat with the next lower contrast level (25%).

10) Continue until the child stops looking toward the card with the "Heidi" Face. The last contrast level the child looks at is presumed to be the lowest level of contrast he or she can see.

BE CONCERNED IF...

- ❑ There is no improvement in contrast sensitivity from previous testing.
- ❑ The child does not respond to the 25% or 10% "Heidi" Low Contrast face.
- ❑ The child does not look at faces and utilize visual communication.

BE PLEASED IF...

Any visual responses are noted in children who do not generally react visually. The child seems to be aware of the low contrast faces.

SUPPRESSION

The visual-processing parts of the infant's brain depend greatly on equally clear, focused images from both eyes. During the first 4 months, this allows the brain to "learn" how to see. If the brain detects that the image from one eye is less clear or discrepant from that of the other eye, it automatically suppresses or turns off the weaker image. If the brain is deprived of or suppresses visual information for some critical period of time, permanent reduction of visual acuity can result. This process is called amblyopia, the most common cause of visual loss in children in the United States (Teplin, S., 1995).

Tavernler stated, "Although estimates vary, the peak of sensitivity for visual development appears to be in the first year of life and to decrease gradually until age 6 (Assaf, 1982; Ingram, 1979; Rogers, Chazan, Fellows, & Tsou, 1982; Von Noorden & Crawford, 1979). These findings indicate that visual stimulation should begin as early as possible, certainly before age 6, preferably within the first months of life (Van de Werfhorst, 1988).

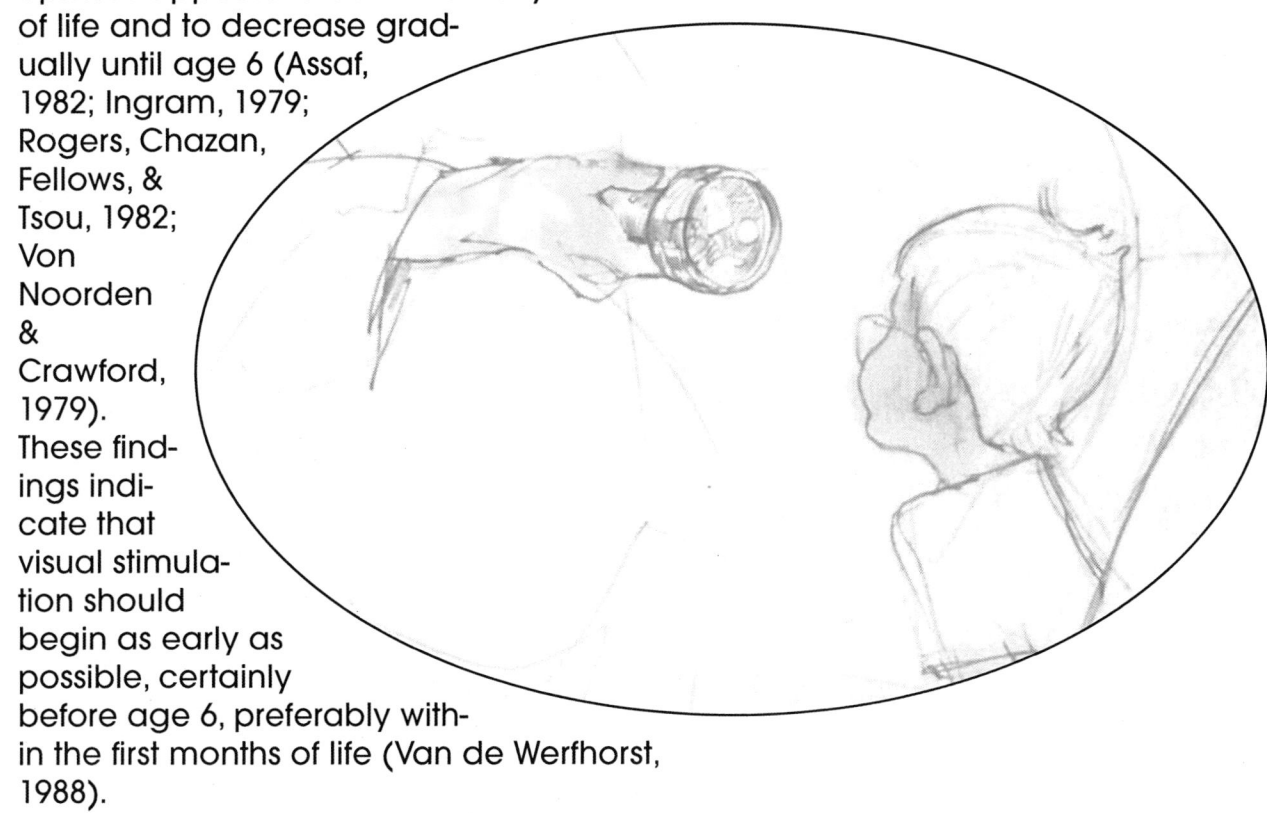

It is extremely important to identify a child who suppresses an eye so visual stimulation can begin quickly. This needs to be done before the age of six years or the eye may not respond to stimulation.

EXPECTED OUTCOMES WHEN COMPARED TO "TYPICAL" VISUAL DEVELOPMENT...

When the child wears the red/green glasses and looks with both eyes at the flashlight from Three Character Flashlight Test he or she should see the red girl, green elephant and the white ball.

PROCEDURE:
1) Use the Three Character Test for children who are functioning at a high enough level to respond.

2) Follow the directions included with the test.

BE CONCERNED IF...
- ❏ Have the child wear the red/green glasses and look with both eyes at the flashlight from Three Character Test.
- ❏ The child sees either the red girl and the white ball only.
- ❏ The child sees the green elephant and white ball only.
- ❏ These examples identify a child who may suppresses an eye.

BE PLEASED IF...
When the child wears the red/green glasses and looks with both eyes at the flashlight from Three Character Test and sees all three of the pictures: red girl, green elephant and white ball.

STEREOPSIS

Binocular vision is the ability of the brain to fuse the separate retinal images into a single image. This ability also makes depth perception easier and is necessary for the finest degree of depth perception. However, lack of binocular vision does not necessarily eliminate the possibility of depth perception... For example, individuals with only monocular vision can still perceive depth from other cues, such as perspective, that is, the learned perception that closer objects appear larger than more distant ones. (Teplin, S., 1995).

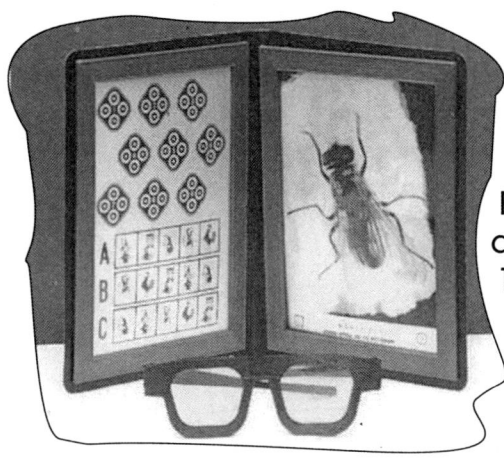

EXPECTED OUTCOMES WHEN COMPARED TO "TYPICAL" VISUAL DEVELOPMENT...
Between 6 and 8 months a baby should see with depth as sharply as most adults (Maurer & Maurer, 1988).

PROCEDURE...

1) Place the child in the best position for comfort and motor stability and head control.

2) Use the Stereo Fly Test with children who have the abilities to respond to the test.

3) Put the Stereo glasses on the child, work fast because some children may try to take them off.

4) Watch the child's face, if he or she has experienced "flyness" you will see a startled face as the wings will pop up if stereo vision is present.

5) If the child is able ask him or her to pick up the wings.

6) If the fingers try to pinch the wings you can assume stereo vision is in place.

7) If the child just touches the stereo wings, stereo is probably not present.

8) If the child can talk he or she will tell you what is seen as this is a motivating test.

9) If this test is too difficult for the child observe him or her at play.

10) Watch to see if the child attempts to look into a can for a toy.

BE CONCERNED IF...
- There is no response to the fly.
- If the child just puts his or her finger on the wings rather than attempting to pick the wings up.
- The child does not attempt to look into the can for a toy.

BE PLEASED IF...
The child's face shows surprise when looking at the fly.

The child tries to pinch the wings when attempting to pick them up.

The child tells you the wings pop up.

The child attempts to look into a can for a toy.

COLOR VISION

Infants are more interested in black and white than color because rods in peripheral vision are more developed than central vision. Research indicates the development of central vision where color is processed occurs around two months of age. (Powell, S. 1996)

"Newborn infants display some degree of colour vision. Adams, Maurer and Davis (1986) reported that newborns differentiated grey from green, from yellow and from red. For each of these colors they preferred to look at colour and grey checkerboards compared to grey squares, matched for overall luminance. However, the newborns showed no evidence of discriminating between grey and blue." By 3 months infants display broadly trichromatic color perception. "Loss of color perception is often irregular in impaired vision; thus color vision tests alone do not depict the loss of function, observations are needed." (Hyvärinen, 1985).

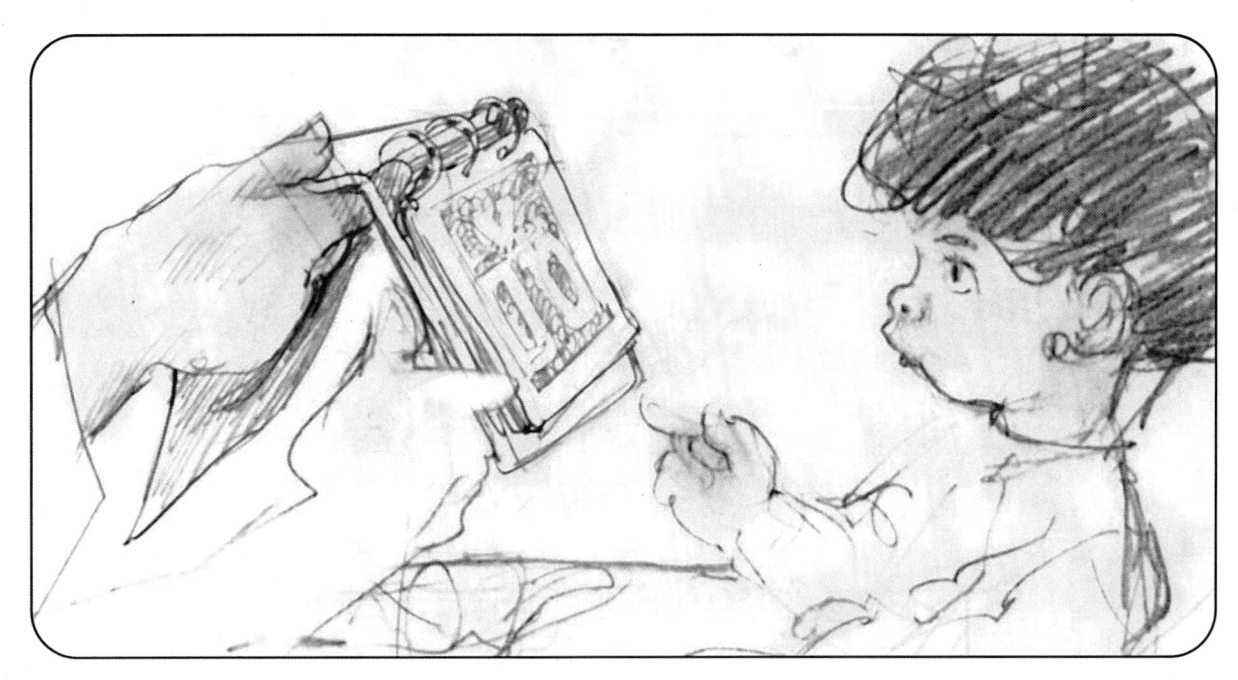

PERCEPTION OF COLOR IS BASED ON 3 DIFFERENT NEURAL FUNCTIONS

1) Absorption of light energy in 3 types of cone cells in various location of the retina.
    L-Cones (long wave length sensitive or red)
    M-Cones (middle wave-length sensitive or green)
    S-Cones (short wave length sensitive or blue)

2) Comparison of the absorption rates in these 3 different cones.

3) Abstraction of color by the cerebral cortex from this comparison. Color perception tests include Ishihara type tests (look like bubbles with a figure merged in the bubbles) and quantitative color vision type tests. Most Ishihara tests are designed to screen for red and green defects and do not pick up acquired defects in the blue-yellow axis. Keep in mind most children with vision

impairments will probably fail an Ishihara red/green screening test. These children need to be tested with quantitative color vision tests that include 15 hues to determine the areas of color confusion.

Color recognition/naming (CR) and color matching (CM) is used in schools as teaching tools to teach concepts such as same and different, grouping items, patterning and even classification. Thus the teacher may think a child doesn't have these concepts when the poor performance may be due to an undiagnosed color deficiency once a color deficit is identified. Teachers can adapt their teaching methods to be less dependent on color discrimination, if necessary.

Keep in mind that children who have color deficits can sometimes match and correctly name colors even though what they see is not true color perception but color recognition. Assessment of a some young children's color functioning can be obtained through observation of their color matching and naming/recognition abilities.

I like to use the red/green screener, **"Color Vision Testing Made Easy Test"**, with children functioning at an 18 month cognitive level in order to screen a child's red/green perception (CP). It can be adapted for children with handicaps such as non-verbal (can point at or place the LEA circle from the **LEA 3-D** Puzzle on the big circle), or non-motor (can eye gaze at big circle).

EXPECTED OUTCOMES WHEN COMPARED TO "TYPICAL" VISUAL DEVELOPMENT...
This area can only be assessed with children who function at least at an 18 – 24 month level. The child was able to match all colors (CM) presented and was able to name or indicate recognition of the color (CR). Child correctly identified 8 of 9 of the Ishihara plates on the **"Color Vision Testing Made Easy Test"** (CP) or passed screening criteria for any other test used.

PROCEDURE:
1) Place child in the best position for comfort motor stability and head control.

2) See if child can match colors utilizing technique appropriate to child's needs (CM).

3) See if the child can name or identify the colors (CR).

4) Follow the test instructions for the," Color Vision Testing Made Easy Test" or what ever Ishihara type test is used (CP).

BE CONCERNED IF...
❑ The child can not pass the Ishihara type red/green screener type tests.
❑ The child can not match (CM) or name or recognize (CR) colors by 2 years of age.
❑ If the child exhibits color confusion in his or her daily life activities.

BE PLEASED IF...
If the child can match and identify color names.
If the child passes the color vision screeners.
If the child does not show color difficulties in his/her daily life.

VISUAL PERCEPTION

EXPECTED OUTCOMES WHEN COMPARED TO TYPICAL VISUAL DEVELOPMENT...

Child exhibits visual perception skills at the development level appropriate for the child.

- ❑ Visual Discrimination (VD)- Awareness of distinctive features of forms including shape, orientation, size and color.

- ❑ Visual Figure-Ground (VFG) - Ability to attend to a specific feature or form while maintaining an awareness of the relationship of this form to the background information.

- ❑ Visual Closure (VC) - Ability to be aware of clues in the visual stimulus that allow determining the final percept with only some of the details present. Visual closure in reading allows us to perceive an entire word accurately when only part of the word is visible.

- ❑ Visual Memory (VM) - Ability to recognize and recall visually presented information. Spelling requires recall of visual information, reading and math require matching the word/number on the page with a stored image.

- ❑ Visual Spatial Relationships (VSR) - The ability to develop normal internal and external spatial concepts used to interact with and organize the environment, make judgements about location of objects and the child's body

- ❑ Visual Form Constancy (VFC) - Ability to recognize that an object has invariant properties such as: shape, position and size even though sensory information received about it has changed. For example, when we see an object as its true shape even when it is seen at an angle relative to our line of sight, i.e., we see a plate as round even if it is held at an angle. The ability to perceiving similarities and differences in geometric figures, symbols, pictures and words.

- ❑ Visual Sequential Memory (VSM) - Ability to observe, recognize, remember, recall and reproduce the sequence of objects, symbols, etc. in whatever means appropriate for the child.

PROCEDURE:
1) It is suggested you utilize the Individualized Systematic Assessment of Visual Perceptual Skills to assess the above areas for infants and multihandicapped children (Langley, 1999).
2) Observe the child as he/she performs tasks.

BE CONCERNED IF...
The child exhibits difficulty in any of the above areas.

BE PLEASED IF...
Age appropriate visual perceptual skills are observed.

APPENDIX A

Scope & Sequence Vision Assessment Tests & Materials

ITEM NAME	PART #	DOMAIN	Birth to 3 yrs	Special Needs	Baby Screen	Play Screen	School Screen
Heidi Doll	1011	Fix/Stim	X	X			
2" Heidi Fix Stick	A2530	Fix/Stim	X	X	X		
5" Heidi Fix Stick	A2531	Fix/Stim	X	X			
8" Heidi Fix Stick	A2532	Fix/Stim	X	X			
LEA Gratings	A2533	Acuity	X	X	X		
Gray Apron	1010	Misc	X	X	X		
LEA Sym 3-D Puzzle	A2516	Stim	X	X		X	
2 Penlights/Caps	1016	Vis Effic	X	X	X	X	X
LEA Playing Card	A2525	Acuity	X	X			
LEA Sym Flash Cards	A2527	Acuity	X	X			
Hiding Heidi L C Face	A2535	Low Con	X	X			
Enhancement Test	A2528	Low Con		X			X
Stimulation Toy		Screening			X	X	
Black on White Bk	2003	Stim	X	X	X	X	
White on Black Bk	2004	Stim	X	X	X	X	
Low Vis Bottle Cover	1018-20	Stim	X	X			
Stereo Fly/Glasses	1027	Stereo		X		X	
Eye Cube	2183	Stereo					X
Random Dot E	1028	Stereo				X	X
3 Char Test	2181	Binoc				X	X
PAIVI Book	1022	Acuity				X	
LEA Single Sym	A2506	Acuity					X
LEA Sym 15 Line	A2501	Acuity					X
MASS Dist Test	A2590	Acuity					X
MASS Near Test	A2589	Acuity					X
LEA Clear-Cuts	2558	Acuity		X			
LEA Sym Near Card	A2508	Acuity					X
Domino Cards	2515	Acuity		X			
Cone Adaptation	A2529	Cone					X
Apple Disp Eye Cover	3103	Occluder				X	X
Color Vis Test Easy	2000	Color				X	X
"Vis Assess of Inf & Special Needs Chldrn"	1026	Book	PART 1	PART 1	PART 2	PART 2	

Tests available from Vision Associates...www.visionkits.com

Vision Associates   www.visionkits.com   K Appleby, M.A.

APPENDIX: B

Parent/Care Taker Interview

| CHILD'S NAME: _____ DOB _____ |
| INTERVIEW DATE: _____ PARENT: _____ |
| AGENCY: _____ HOME ADDRESS _____ |
| COMPLETED BY: _____ _____ |
| _____ _____ |
| _____ PHONE: _____ |

PREMATURE? __YES __NO   MEDICATIONS? __YES __NO   SEIZURES? __YES __NO

Does anyone in the child's biological family have vision problems or wear glasses? __Yes __No

If so, what are the vision problems?

Has the child been evaluated by an eye doctor? ___Yes ___No ___ If so, when?_____

Was the doctor an ophthalmologist? ___Yes ___No,   An optometrist? ___Yes No___

Where glasses prescribed? ___Yes ___No,   If so, what for: ___distance ___ near?

Does the child tolerate the glasses? ___Yes ___No ___N/A, Is child light sensitive? ___Yes ___No___

When are you to go back to see the doctor?_____

What did you learn from the doctor visit?

Do you agree with the doctor's interpretation of the child's visual condition? ___Yes ___No

Do you still have questions about the child's vision? ___Yes ___No, If so, what are they?

What does the child do that seems unusual as related to the use of vision?

What does the child do indicating the possibility of a visual response?

APPENDIX C

"TYPICAL" VISUAL DEVELOPMENT...

In order to assess vision you will need to review visual development of children who are developing typically so you can identify deviations from typical development. The following chart can be used as a guide. In some cases you may not be looking for deviations but for any signs of vision.

VISUAL DEVELOPMENT OF "TYPICALLY" DEVELOPING CHILDREN

AGE   **BEHAVIOR**

Birth - 1 month
- __Turns eyes & head to look at light sources
- __Appears to look through rather than at people
- __Black & white (high contrast) objects most interesting
- __PUPILS RESPOND TO LIGHT may be constricted 1st few weeks
- __FIXATION noted as child nurses with open eyes
- __MUSCLE BALANCE eye turn may be present, aligning later
- __HORIZONTAL PURSUITS with head movement, may be jerky
- __VERTICAL PURSUITS emerging
- __SHIFT OF GAZE from toy to toy slow with head movement
- __ACUITY poor due to immaturity of retina
- __CONTRAST SENSITIVITY poor due to immaturity of retina

2-3 months
- __Social smile by 3 months
- __Reaches toward & later grasps hanging objects.
- __FIXATION intense eye contact, interest in looking at moving lips
- __VERTICAL/HORIZONTAL PURSUITS with eyes only.
- __PERIPHERAL VISUAL RESPONSES within 60°
- __COLOR VISION prefers colored toys to black & white
- __ACCOMMODATES to different distances by 3 months
- __STEREOPSIS by 3 months

4 - 6 months
- __First time watching own hands is noted
- __Reaches toward faces & objects
- __Watches toys fall or roll away
- __VISUAL SPHERE gradually extends outward
- __SHIFT OF GAZE across midline
- __CONVERGENCE present by 6 months
- __PERIPHERAL VISUAL FIELDS responses within 180°
- __ACUITY recognizes distance objects, watches his or her hands.

7-10 months
- __Interest in pictures in books
- __Recognizes partially hidden objects
- __Pictures in books become interesting
- __FIXATION eye hand coordination improving
- __PERIPHERAL VISION symmetrical
- __ACUITY notices small objects like cereal & crumbs
- __PERCEPTION develops perception to form & size

11-12 months
- __Looks through window
- __Recognizes people, objects and pictures
- __Likes to play Peek-a-book
- __DEPTH PERCEPTION explores depth by looking into containers
- __COLOR PERCEPTION full color vision.

Vision Associates   www.visionkits.com   K. Appleby, M.A.

APPENDIX D

CHARACTERISTICS OF CEREBRAL VISUAL IMPAIRMENT CHECKLIST
Children with other types of visual impairments may exhibit some of these characteristics.

CHILD'S NAME_____ AGE_____ DATE_____ RESPONDENT'S NAME &
RELATION TO CHILD_____ A child may be suspected
of having a cerebral visual loss when extent of visual loss is unexplained by ocular
abnormalities. Etiologies may include cerebral palsy, asphyxia, intracerebral hemor-

Please check any areas below that pertain to the child.

APPEARANCE
___Does not look blind
___Blank facial expression
___Lack of visual communication skills
___Eye movements smooth, but aimless
___Nystagmus (rapid eye movement) rarely seen

VISION FUNCTION
___Visual function varies from day to day or hour to hour
___Limited visual attention and lacks visual curiosity
___Aware of distant objects, but not able to identify
___Spontaneous visual activity has short duration
___Visual learning tiring
___Closes eyes while listening
___Balance improved with eyes closed
___Look away from people and objects
___Consistently look to either side when visual looking
___When visually reaching looks with a slight downward gaze
___Turns head to side when reaching, as if using peripheral fields
___Uses touch to identify objects

MOBILITY SKILLS
___Occasionally "sees" better traveling in a car
___Difficulties with depth perception, inaccurate reach
___Unable to estimate distances
___Difficulties with spatial interpretation
___Avoids obstacles, but unable to use vision for close work

IMPROVED VISUAL PERFORMANCE
___When in familiar environments and when using familiar objects
___When told "what" to look for and "where" to look
___When objects are held close to eyes when viewing
___When objects are widely spaced
___When looking at one object verses a group of objects
___When color is used to assist in identification of objects or shapes
___When objects are against a plain background & paired with movement & sound

Adapted: Jan, J., Groenveld, A., Sykanda, A., Hoyt, C. (1987)
Vision Associates   www.visionkits.com

APPENDIX: E

INFANTS & CHILDREN with SPECIAL NEEDS Vision Assessment
Recording Form
by Kathleen Appleby, M.A.

CHILD'S NAME:_____ DOB_____ TEST DATE_____ PARENT_____
AGENCY/ADDRESS_____ HOME ADDRESS_____

PHONE_____ PHONE:_____

MEDICAL INFORMATION: Dr's visual diagnosis_____
Legally Blind: ___yes ___no , Complete to explain legally blind criteria: Field Deficits_____
Distance Acuity (right) _____/Corrected_____, Distance Acuity (left) _____/Corrected_____
Near Acuity (right)_____/Corrected_____, Near Acuity (left)_____/Corrected_____
Visually Functions as if legally Blind ___yes ___no, Performance indicates possibility of CVI ___yes ___no
Glasses prescribed: ___yes ___no (if yes): ___worn ___not worn ___does not like to wear them

1. OBSERVATION & INTERVIEW (check all that apply)
Premature? ___yes___no , if yes gestation/wks_____ Medication(s):_____
Mode of Communication_____ Best position & time to assess_____
___Head tilt/turn ___droopy eyelid ___Holds items close to eyes ___Nystagmus/rapid eye mvmnt
___Abnormal appearance to eyes ___Unusual eye(s) position
<u>REACTIONS TO LIGHT:</u>
___turns to light ___avoids light ___reaches for light ___quiets to lighting changes
<u>OFTEN SEEN IN CHILDREN WITH CORTICAL/CEREBRAL VISION PROBLEMS:</u>
___Lacks interest in looking
___Visual responses fluctuate day to day
___Tends to look away from people and objects
___Smooth, aimless eye movements
___Responds best when objects placed peripherally
___Visual attention best to objects in motion
___Quick side to side head movement when looking
___Hand searching movements when locating items
<u>EARLY VISUAL MILESTONES:</u>
___Eye contact ___Hand regard ___Hands to midline ___Visual Communication
___Visual Guided Reach ___Response within 10' to people ___Normal turning to sounds
___Visually guided crawling/scooting
Notes:

2. PUPILLARY RESPONSES TO PENLIGHT (Do Not Complete If Seizure Prone or if on Medication)
Normal pupillary responses include pupils constricting in bright light and dilating in dim light.
<u>Direct Response</u> (light in each eye) constriction observed in: ___right ___left
<u>Consensual Response</u> (hand at bridge of nose) constriction observed in: ___right ___left
Notes:

3. VISUAL SPHERE
This is the space within which the child visually responds to motivating objects.
Large object size:___inches   Distance loses visual interest:___
Smallest size: ___inches, Distance loses visual interest:___
For visual response to occur, these stimuli had to be paired with object:: ___sound ___motion
___plain background ___good contrast ___color, Preferred: color_____ & object_____
Notes:

4. FIXATION
Do not cover an eye, place a motivating toy at eye level, 18" from nose & note eye positions:
R: ___central ___out ___in _____other, L: ___central ___out ___in _____other
If needed use a slant board, magnet & metal objects to elicit fixation. Note fixation with:
Both eyes: ___size ___duration,   R: ___size ___duration, L: ___size ___duration
Note unusual head & eye positions:_____
Notes:

5. MUSCLE BALANCE
Hirschberg (direct penlight reflection): (R) ___central ___out ___in,   (L) ___central ___out ___in
Alternate Cover Movement: (R) ___in to out ___out to in, (L) ___in to out ___out to in
Cover/Uncover: eye turn (R) ___in ___out ___no turn   (L) ___in ___out, ___no turn

Child's Right   Child's Left
Eyes as you look at child

Notes:

6. OCULAR PURSUITS
Visually follow a moving object in an arc at eye level, 18" from child's eyes. Check results below.

	Smooth	Jerky	Brk Fix	Brk/Midline	Latency of mvm
Horizontal:					
Vertical:					
Diagonal:					

___eye mvnt only ___head & eye mvnt ___head   still when asked ___head needed to be held
___improved w/pointing, Eyes able to get in all positions of gaze when head still: ___yes ___no
Notes:

7. NEAR POINT OF CONVERGENCE
When object (held 18" from bridge of nose at eye level) moves slowly toward bridge of nose, eyes should move smoothly and equally to about 3-4" from nose.
Deviating eye: ____right ____left Distance deviated at:_____ Distance recovered_____
Notes:

8. SACCADES/SHIFT OF GAZE (Check the areas the child successfully performed)

BOTH EYES	from midline to right ___	from midline to left ___
"	from eye level up ___	from eye level down ___
"	across midline R to L ___	across midline L to R ___
RIGHT EYE	from midline to right ___	from midline to left ___
"	from eye level up ___	from eye level down ___
"	across midline R to L ___	across midline L to R ___
LEFT EYE	from midline to right ___	from midline to left ___
"	from eye level up ___	from eye level down ___
"	across midline R to L ___	across midline L to R ___

Notes:

9. VISUAL FIELD

Peripheral Vision
Side view   Top View

Peripheral Field Limitations	Right	Left	Upper	Lower
Delayed Response				

Notes (including any central visual fields observations):

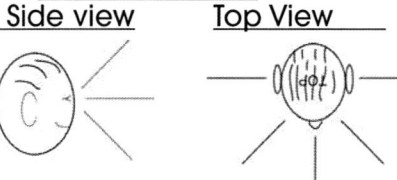

Put an "X" at point head turned to light

10. ACUITY

A) Functional Acuity
When functional objects are used, list: "size of target" & furthest distance

Near	(both)	size	distance	(right)	size	distance	(left)	size	distance
Distance:	(both)	size	distance	(right)	size	distance	(left)	size	distance

Near object Used _____ Distance object used _____

B) Grating Acuity
Present a striped pattern in front of the child simultaneously with a gray surface. The striped pattern is more interesting to look at then the gray surface. Continue presenting the gratings of decreasing widths. When the child stops responding to the gratings it is most likely because he/she can no longer detect the presence of the parallel lines as they blur to gray. Report size of last grating the child responded to and how far away it was.

LEA Grating Paddles
Check narrowest stripes to which child responds & furthest distance at which he/she responds.

Both eyes: (cpcm)	0.25	0.5	1.0	2.0	4.0	8.0	Distance away ___
Right eye: (cpcm)	0.25	0.5	1.0	2.0	4.0	8.	Distance away ___
Left eye: (cpcm)	0.25	0.5	1.0	2.0	4.0	8.0	Distance away ___

C) Optotype Acuity

Near:	(both) 20/___	(right) 20/___	(left) 20/___	Test Used ___
Distance:	(both) 20/___	(right) 20/___	(left) 20/___	Test Used ___

11) CONTRAST SENSITIVITY
Check the lowest contrast level to which the child responds.

	"Hiding Heidi" reaction to Contrast Level					Furthest Distance Responds to Heidi		Lighting Needs		
Both	100%	25%	10%	5%	1.25%	inches	feet	high	med	low
Right	100%	25%	10%	5%	1.25%	inches	feet	high	med	low
Left	100%	25%	10%	5%	1.25%	inches	feet	high	med	low

Notes:

12. SUPPRESSION
Appears to suppress: ___right eye, ___left eye, ___did not try
Test Used_____

Notes:

13. STEREOPSIS/DEPTH PERCEPTION
Demonstrates depth perception: ___yes, ___no ___did not assess ___

Notes:

14. COLOR VISION RED/GREEN SCREENING
Ishihara type screens for red/green. Responded by: ___pointing ___matching ___naming
Responses indicate: ___normal ___confused ___possible defect
Test used:_____

Notes:

15. VISION PRECEPTION
Questionable performance: ___VD   ___VFG   ___VC   ___VM   ___VSR   ___VFC   ___VSM

Notes:

SUMMARY RESULTS
Unusual responses noted in the following areas (check all that apply):
___Observations ___Pupillary Resp ___Visual Sphere ___Fixation ___Muscle Balance
___Ocular Pursuits ___Convergence ___Shift of Gaze ___Visual Fields ___Acuity
___Contrast Sens ___Suppression ___Stereopsis ___Color Red/Green
___Visual Perception
Refer to:_____

COMMENTS & SUGGESTIONS: (Attach additional pages, if necessary.)

Examiner_____
Date_____
Address_____
_____
Phone _____

APPENDIX: F

BABIES & CHILDREN With "SPECIAL NEEDS"
Vision Assessment
Reporting Form
by Kathleen Appleby, M.A.

CHILD'S NAME:_____ DOB_____ TEST DATE:_____ PARENT: _____
AGENCY/ADDRESS_____ HOME ADDRESS _____
_____ _____
_____ _____
PHONE_____ PHONE:_____

MEDICAL INFORMATION:

Dr's Visual Diagnosis &
Treatment_____
_____

Legally Blind: __yes __no, Field Deficits: (RE) __yes __no, (LE) __yes __no, Degree of Loss_____
RIGHT EYE: Dist Acuity ____/Corrected____, Near Acuity ____/Corrected____ Patching: __yes __no
LEFT EYE: Dist Acuity ____/Corrected____, Near Acuity ____/Corrected____ Patching: __yes __no
Visually functions as if legally Blind: __yes __no, Medical history indicates possibility of CVI: __yes __no
Glasses Prescribed: __yes __no   (if yes): __worn __not worn __resists glasses __resists patch
Premature: __yes __no (if yes): ____gestation/wks ___weight _____medical considerations
Mode of Communication: Best position/time to assess

This vision assessment measures performance and does not replace a doctor's examination. Non-visual factors may affect performance, such as motor abilities, processing skills, cooperation and cognitive abilities.

OBSERVATION & INTERVIEW

Visual functioning is more than the sum of the components of a vision assessment. It is important to observe the child's everyday activities in order to gain insights into how he or she uses vision. Lighting conditions for best visual response: __low __medium __high, Color preference: _____

__Red Flag   __OK   __unusual

COMMENTS:

PUPILLARY RESPONSES

The child's state of alertness, attentiveness and reaction to medications can influence pupil size. Normal pupillary responses include pupils getting smaller in bright light and getting bigger in dim light. If the child is on medication, is light sensitive, or seizure prone do not complete this area.

___on medications   ___seizure prone

___Red Flag   ___OK Response   ___unable to determine   ___did not try

COMMENTS:

VISUAL SPHERE & VISUAL ATTENTION

VISUAL SPHERE is the space within which a child looks at interesting visual objects of certain size, color, contrast and speed of movement. We need to discover the child's visual sphere so we know where to present toys and ourselves.

Distance loses interest in looking_____, Smallest object looked at before losing interest_____, Object most interested in_____, In order for the child to look at an object it is necessary to pair it with: ___sound,   ___movement,   ___plain background,   ___good contrast

___Red Flag   ___OK response   ___Emerging   ___Unable to determine   ___did not try

COMMENTS:

FIXATION/ABILITY TO LOOK AT AN OBJECT

A child's ability to look at an object on the best viewing part of the eye is FIXATION. It is important to determine: which eye is used, if each eye alternates fixation to look at a toy, how close child gets and if a head turn is used for close looking. If responses appear unusual the assessment will attempt to look for a reason.

___Red Flag   ___OK response   ___Emerging   ___Unable to determine   ___did not try

COMMENTS:

MUSCLE BALANCE/EYE POSITIONS

Each eye is controlled by six muscles that position the eyes without either eye turning in, out, up or down. When there is a muscle imbalance a child may have trouble seeing one clear image.

___Red Flag   ___OK response   ___unable to determine   ___did not try

COMMENTS:

OCULAR PURSUITS/VISUALLY FOLLOWING MOVING OBJECTS

By one year of age a child should be able to visually follow a moving toy with smooth eye movements as it moves sideways, up and down, diagonally and in a circle (OCULAR PURSUITS). A child should be able to do this without head movement when objects are moved in the center of the visual field.
___eye movement only ___head+eye movement ___head still when asked ___head had to be held ___improved with pointing, Eyes able to get in all positions of gaze when head still: ___yes ___no

___Red Flag   ___OK response   ___Emerging   ___unable to determine   ___did not try

COMMENTS:

CONVERGENCE/MOVEMENT OF BOTH EYES INWARD

This is related to the ability of the brain to unite the image of an object, created in each eye, into a single image. The child looks at an interesting toy as it moves closer (NEAR POINT OF CONVERGENCE). By 6 mos of age the eyes should turn in equally and smoothly as toy gets to about 3" from the child's nose.

___Red Flag   ___OK response   ___unable to determine   ___did not try

COMMENTS:

SACCADES/SHIFT OF GAZE

The child should be able to shift looking from one toy to another when the toys are placed in a variety of places.
Shift gaze (SACCADES) abilities are necessary to easily copy from book to paper, shift gaze to find objects on a page or at distance, etc.

___**Red Flag**   ___OK response   ___Emerging   ___Unable to determine   ___did not try

COMMENTS:

VISUAL FIELDS

Peripheral vision (side vision) is the range of space visible to the child's eye as he/she looks straight ahead. It gives the child information about the outline and shade of surroundings and offers cues when something appears from the side. It is measured by seeing how far a toy, coming from the side, has to be moved toward the child's midline before it is noticed. Central visual fields can be informally assessed in a play situation.

___**Red Flag**   ___OK central   ___OK Peripheral   ___unable to determine   ___did not try

COMMENTS:

ACUITY

Acuity is the ability of the eyes to discern details. Near acuity measures the ability to see at a near range. Distance acuity measures the ability to see at a distance. Acuity in a young child can be tested with black & white stripes (gratings), real objects (functional), black & white symbols, or letters or numbers (optotypes).

___**Red Flag** __near __distance __functional __grating __optotype __unable to determine __didn't try

COMMENTS:

CONTRAST SENSITIVITY

Contrast sensitivity is the ability to see objects of low contrast. Being able to see at low contrast is important in visual communication. A child with poor contrast sensitivity may have problems seeing face details and may lose important communicative information. Wearing bright lipstick and eyeliner improves contrast.

___**Red Flag**   ___OK response   ___unable to determine   ___did not try

COMMENTS:

SUPPRESSION OF AN EYE/BINOCULARITY

Subconscious inhibition of input from one eye due to several causes, usually associated with strabismus (eye turn) and amblyopia (deceased vision in one eye unexplained by refractive error or observable eye disease).

___**Red Flag**   ___right   ___left   ___OK response   ___unable to determine   ___didn't try

COMMENTS:

STEREOPSIS/DEPTH PERCEPTION

Binocular depth perception which is the visual blending of two similar but not identical images (one falling on each retina) into one, with resulting visual perception of solidity and depth.

___**Red Flag**   ___OK response   ___unable to determine   ___did not try

COMMENTS:

COLOR VISION SCREENING FOR RED/GREEN

<u>Color vision perception</u> (CVP) screenings for red green attempt to identify possible problems in the red or green signaling mechanism. This is not the same as <u>*color recognition*</u> (CR) (the ability to correctly name colors) or _ (CM) (the ability to match colors). Color vision perception difficulties can impair learning at critical ages of educational development.

__Red Flag (CVP)   __OK response   __unable to determine   __did not try
__Red Flag (CR)   __OK response   __unable to determine   __did not try
__Red Flag (CM)   __OK response   __unable to determine   __did not try

COMMENTS:

VISION PERCEPTION

One of the most important characteristics of visual perception is that it is organized: we perceive a world of objects, people and events, which move and change in a unified, coherent fashion.

__**Red Flag** Informal observations indicated questionable performance in the following areas:
   __VD   __VFG   __VC   __VM   __VSR   __VFC   __VSM

COMMENTS:

SUMMARY

The child exhibited **Red Flags** in the following areas:

__Observations	__Pupillary Responses	__Visual Sphere	__Fixation
__Muscle Balance	__Ocular Pursuits	__Near Pt Convergence	__Shift of Gaze
__Visual Fields	__Acuity	__Contrast Sensitivity	__Suppression
__Stereopsis	__Color Red/Green	__Poor Visual Perception	

RECOMMENDATIONS/SUGGESTIONS

APPENDIX: G

REFERENCES
CORTICAL/CEREBRAL VISUAL IMPAIRMENT

Alexander, P.K. The effects of brain damage on visual functioning in children. Journal of Visual Impairment and Blindness, September 1990. 84(7), 372-376.

Balliet, R. and others. Visual field rehabilitation in the cortically blind? Journal of Neurology, Neurosurgery and Psychiatry. 1985, 48, 1113-1124.

Birch, Eileen E. and others. Forced choice preferential looking acuity of children with cortical visual impairment. Developmental Medicine and Child Neurology, August 1991, 33(8).

Burgess, P., Johnson, A., Ocular defects in Infants of extremely low birth weight and low gestational age. British Journal of Ophthalmology, February 1991, 75(2), 84-87.

Dale, W.F., Brain pathology and blindness: special considerations. Journal of Visual Impairment and Blindness, October 1981, 75(8), 313-316.

Eken, P., and others. Relation between neonatal cranial ultrasound abnormalities and cerebral visual impairment in infancy. Developmental Medicine and Child Neurology, January 1994, 36(1), 3-15.

Erin, J., (1989) Cortical Visual impairment: implications for service delivery. Journal of Vision Rehabilitation. Vol. 3, No. 4, pp 1-10.

Foley, J. Central visual disturbances. Developmental Medicine & Child Neurology, February 1987, 29(1), 116-120.

Foley, J., Gordon, N. Recovery from cortical blindness. Developmental Medicine & Child Neurology, June 1985, 27(3), 383-387.

Frank, Y., and others. Flash and pattern-reversal visual evoked potential abnormalities in infants and children with cerebral blindness. Developmental Medicine and child Neurology, April 1992, 34(4), 305-315.

Gianutsos, R., Ramsey, G., Enabling rehabilitation optometrists to help survivors of acquired brain injury. Journal of Vision Rehabilitation, January, 1988, 2(1), 37-58.

Groenendall, F., Hof-van D., Jacki van. Visual deficits and improvements in children after perinatal hypoxia. Journal of Visual Impairment and Blindness, May 1992, 86(5), 215-218.

Hof-van Duin, J. van and Mohn, G. Optokinetic and spontaneous nystagmus in children with neurological disorders. Behavioural Brain Research, 1983, 10, 163-175.

Hoyt, C.S., Neurovisual adaptations to subnormal vision in children. In Insight in sight: proceedings of the fifth Canadian interdisciplinary conference on the visually impaired child, Vancouver, 1984, 102-113.

Groenveld, M., Characteristics and needs of children with cortical visual impairment. 1-12.

Jan, J., Groenveld, M., (1980) Observations on the habilitation of children with cortical visual impairment, Journal of Visual Impairment and Blindness, January 1990, 11-15.

Jan, J., Groenveld, M., Visual behaviour and adaptations associated with cortical and ocular impairments in children. Journal of Visual Impairment and Blindness, April 1993, 87(4), 101-105.

Jan, E., Groenveld, M., Sykanda, A.M., C.S. Hoyt, Behavioural characteristics of children with permanent cortical visual impairment. Developmental Medicine and Child Neurology, October 1987, 29(5), 571-576.

Jan, J., Robinson, G., Scott, E., A multidisciplinary approach to the problems of the multi-handicapped blind child. CMA Journal, October 1973, Vol. 109, 705-707.

Jan, J., Robinson, Geoffrey, G., A Multidisciplinary Program for visually impaired children and youths. International Ophthalmology Clinics, Spring 1989, Vol 29 No 1.

Jan, J., Whiting, S., Wong, P., Flodmark, O., Farrell, K., McCormick, A., (1985) Permanent cortical visual impairment In children. Developmental Medicine & Child Neurology, 27, 730-739.

Jan, J., and others, Photophobia and cortical visual impairment. Developmental Medicine and Child Neurology, Jun 1993, 35(6), 473-477.

Lambert, S., Hoyt, C., Jan, J., Barkovich, J., Flodmark, G., Visual recovery from hypoxic cortical blindness during childhood. Arch Ophthalmology, Vol 1095, Oct 1987, 1371-1377.

Kupersmith, N., Nelson, J., Preserved visual evoked potential in infancy cortical blindness. Neuro-ophthalmology, 1986, 6(2), 85-94.

Mancini, J. and others, Face recognition in children with early right or left brain damage. Developmental Medicine and Child Neurology, February 1993, 36(2), 156-166.

McCulloch, D.L., Taylor, N.J. Cortical blindness in children: utility of flash VEPs". Pediatric Neurology. 1992. Mar-Apr, 8(2) 156.

Morse, M., Cortical visual impairment in young children with multiple disabilities. Journal of Visual Impairment and Blindness, May 1990, 84(5), 200-203.

Roland, El, Jan, J., Hill, A., Wong, K., Cortical visual impairment following birth asphyxia. Pediatric Neurology, May-June 1996, Vol. 2: No. 3, 133-137.

Whiting, S. and others, Permanent cortical visual impairment in children. Developmental Medicine and Child Neurology, December 1985, 27(6), 730-739.

APPENDIX H
BIBLIOGRAPHY

American Academy of Ophthalmology Policy Statement: #812 "Infant/Child Vision Screening", Approved by the American Academy of Ophthalmology., September, 1996.

Bradley, A. and Freeman, R.D. (1982). Contrast sensitivity in children. Vision Research, 22, 953-959.

Brown, D., (2001). Follow the Child-Approaches to Assessing the Function Vision and Hearing of Young Children with Congenital Deaf-Blindness. California Deaf-Blind Services reSources, Vol. 10, Number 9, 1-3.

Cassin, B., Solomon, S., Rubin, M. (1990). Dictionary of Eye Terminology. Gainesville, Florida: Triad Publishing Co.

Good, W.V., & Hoyt, C.S. (1989). Behavioral correlates of poor vision in children. International Ophthalmology Clinics, 29, 57-60.

Haith, M.M. (1986). Sensory and perceptual processes in early infancy. Journal of Pediatrics, 109, 158-171.

Hoyt, C. Nickel, Bl, & Billson, F. (1982). Ophthalmological examination of the infant. Developmental aspects. Survey of Ophthalmology, 26, 177-185.

Hyvärinen, L. (1994). Assessment of visually impaired infants. Ophthalmology Clinics of North America, 7, 219-225.

Hyvärinen, L. Effect of Visual Impairment on Early Development in Hyvärinen L., BjÖrkman J., Lindquist O. and StenstrÖm I., SynbedÖmning av barn och ungdomar på tidig utvecklingsnivå (available also as an article obtained from Vision Associates)

Hyvärinen, L. (1988). Vision in children normal and abnormal. Meaford, Ontario: Canadian Deaf-Blind & Rubella Association.

Hyvärinen, L., & Appleby, K. (1996). Visual assessment of infants and children with multi-handicaps. Orlando, FL: Vision Associates.

Hyvärinen L., Bull Soc Belge Ophthalmology 1985, 215:1-16.

Hyvärinen, L (1998) Home page at http://www.lea-test.sgic.fi

Hyvärinen, L (2000) "LH-Materials 2001", CD, Lea-Test Ltd, Helsinki, Vision Associates, FL

Lueck Hall, A., Chen, D., & Kekelis, L. (1997). Developmental guidelines for infants with visual impairment. Louisville, KY: American Printing House for the Blind, Inc.

Martin LJ. The pupil. In Isenberg SJ, ed. The eye in infancy. Chicago: Year Book Medical Publishers, 1989;362.

Mohn, G, & Van Hof-van Duin, J.V.(1986). Development of the binocular and monocular visual fields of human infants during the first year of like. Clinical Vision Science, 1, 51-64.

Norcia, A.M., Tyler, C.W. and Hamer, R.D. (1990). Development of contrast sensitivity in the human infant. Vision Research, 30, 1475-1486.

Optometric Clinical Practice Guidelines for the : #CPG2 "Pediatric Eye and Vision Examination", Approved by the AOA Board of Trustees, June 23, 1994.

Racanelli, R., Vision assessment of the multiply impaired, March 1, 1996 Illinois Vision Conference, Naperville, IL.

Richards, R. (1984) Visual Skills Appraisal. Navato, CA, Academic Therapy Publications.

Riordan-Eva P. Special subjects of pediatric interest. In Vaughn D, Asbury T, Tabbara KF, eds. General ophthalmology, 12th ed. Norwalk, Conn.: Appleton and Lange, 1989; 330.

Powell, S.A., (1996) Neural-based visual stimulation with infants with cortical impairment, Journal of Visual Impairments & Blindness, Sept-Oct 1996, 445-448.

Tavernler, G., (1995) The improvement of vision by visual stimulation and training: A review of the literature, Journal of Visual Impairments & Blindness, May 1995, 143-147.

Teplin, S, (1995) Visual impairment in infants and young children. Infants and Young Children, July 1995.

Thompson, C. (1993) Assessment of child vision and refractive error, Visual Problems in Childhood, Butterworth-Heinemann Ltd., Linacre House, Jordan Hill, Oxford OX28DP.

REFERENCES for Visual Resolution & Health of the Eye

Cassin, B., Solomon, S., Rubin, M. (1990). Dictionary of Eye Terminology. Gainesville, Florida: Triad Publishing Co.

Hyvärinen, L,.(1997), Cone Adaptation Test #2529, Instructional Manual For Vision Testing Products, LaSalle, IL, Precision Vision.

Hyvärinen, L,.(2000), Glossary, http://med-aapos.bu.edu/leaweb/glossar2.html.

Scheiman, M., (1997), Understanding and Managing Vision Deficits: A guide for Occupational Therapists. Thorofare, NJ: Slack, Inc.

Patel, S., and Buckingham, T. (1993), Colour vision assessment in children, Visual Problems in Children, London: Butterworth-Heinemann Ltd.

Zambone A. M., (1989). Serving the young child with visual impairments: An overview of disability impact and intervention needs. In Young Children, 2(2): 11-23.

REFERENCES for Welcome Aboard: An Introduction Letter

American Academy of Ophthalmology Policy Statement: #812 "Infant/Child Vision Screening", Approved by the American Academy of Ophthalmology., September, 1996.

First Look Vision Evaluation and Assessment for Infants, Toddlers, and Preschoolers, Birth through Five Years of Age. California Department of Education, 1998.

Langley, M.B., ISAVE Individualized Systematic Assessment of Visual Efficiency, APH, 1998.

Optometric Clinical Practice Guidelines for the: #CPG2 "Pediatric Eye and Vision Examination", Approved by the AOA Board of Trustees, June 23, 1994.

REFERENCES for the Visual System

Hyvärinen, L (2000) "LH-Materials 2001", CD, Lea-Test Ltd, Helsinki, Vision Associates, FL

REFERENCE for Visual Pathways

Groenveld, M., "Characteristics and Needs of Children with Cortical Visual Impairment", Vancouver, BC.

Hyvärinen, L (2000) "LH-Materials 2001", CD, Lea-Test Ltd, Helsinki, Vision Associates, FL

Scheiman, M., (1997), Understanding and Managing Vision Deficits: A Guide of Occupational Therapists. Thorofare, NJ: Slack, Inc.

REFERENCES for Visual Efficiency

Cassin, B., Solomon, S., Rubin, M. (1990). Dictionary of Eye Terminology. Gainesville, Florida: Triad Publishing Co.
Racanelli, V., (1996), Vision assessment of the multiply impaired, unpublished paper presented at the Illinois Vision Conference, Naperville, IL

Scharre, J., (1995), Functional Vision Issues, unpublished paper presented at Du Page Easter Seals, Rosalie Dold Symposium, DuPage, IL. http://www.uic.edu/~politano/func-vision.HTM

Scheiman, M., (1997), Understanding and Managing Vision Deficits: A guide for Occupational Therapists. Thorofare, NJ: Slack, Inc

REFERENCES for Visual Perception

ESSE 506 MCTP, (2001), Special Needs Children in the General Classroom-Notetaking

Gardner, M., (1997), Test of Visual-Perceptual Skills, Hydesville, CA: Psychological and Educational Pub., Inc.

Guide Chapter 6, http://www.odu.edu/webroot/orgs/Educ/Misc/MCTP.

Langley, M.B., ISAVE Individualized Systematic Assessment of Visual Efficiency, APH, 1998.

Scheiman, M., (1997), Understanding and Managing Vision Deficits: A guide for Occupational Therapists. Thorofare, NJ: Slack, Inc.

REFERENCES Visual Development of "typically" Developing Children & "Non-Typical"

Canadian Deaf-Blind and Rubella Associates, Ontario Canada, Vision screening in pre-school age children.
Hyvärinen, L., Assessment of visually impaired infants, (1994) Ophthalmology Clinics of North American, Vol. 7:2.

Hyvärinen, L., Vision in children normal and abnormal. (1988) Canadian Deaf-Blind and Rubella Associates

Teplin, S.W. (1995), Visual impairment in infants and young children, Infants and young children: An interdisciplinary journal of special care practices. 8, 18-45.

REFERENCE for Cortical/Cerebral Vision Impairment

Jan, J., Groenveld, M., (1980) "Observations on the Habilitation of Children with Cortical Visual Impairment", Journal of Visual Impairment & Blindness, January 1990, 11-15.
H 4-5
Jan, J.E., Groenveld, M., (1993), Visual behaviors and adaptations associated with cortical and ocular impairment in children, Journal of Visual Impairment & Blindness, April, 1993, 101-105.

Jan, J., Whiting, S., Wong, P., Flodmark, O., Farrell, K., McCormick, A., (1985) "Permanent Cortical Visual Impairment In Children"/ Developmental Medicine & Child Neurology, 27, 730-739.

Hyvärinen, L., (2000) "LH-Materials 2001", CD, Lea-Test Ltd, Helsinki

Teplin, S.W. (1995), Visual impairment in infants and young children, Infants and young children: An interdisciplinary journal of special care practices. 8, 18-45.

REFERENCES for Characteristics of Cerebral/Cortical Visual Impairment Checklist

Jan, J.E., Groenveld, A., Sykanda, A.M., Hoyt, C.S. (1987) "Behavioral Characteristics of Children with Permanent Cortical Visual Impairment." Developmental Medicine & Child Neurology, 25,755-762.

REFERENCES for Understanding Behaviors as they Relate to Vision in the Child with C/CVI

Steendam, M., (1989), Cortical Visual Impairment In Children, Royal Blind Society of N.S.W.

REFERENCES for Before You Assess

Begley, S., How to build a baby's brain, Newsweek, Spring/Summer, 1997, 28-32.

Hyvärinen,L. Effect of Visual Impairment on Early Development in Hyvärinen L., BjÖrkman J., Lindquist O. and StenstrÖm I., SynbedÖmning av barn och ungdomar på tidig utvecklingsnivå

Hyvärinen, L. (1994). Assessment of visually impaired infants. Ophthalmology Clinics of North America, 7, 219-225.

Zambone A. M., (1989). Serving the young child with visual impairments: An overview of disability impact and intervention needs. In Young Children, 2(2): 11-23.

VISION SCREENING

BABIES with PLAY
PART 2

by Kathleen Appleby, MA

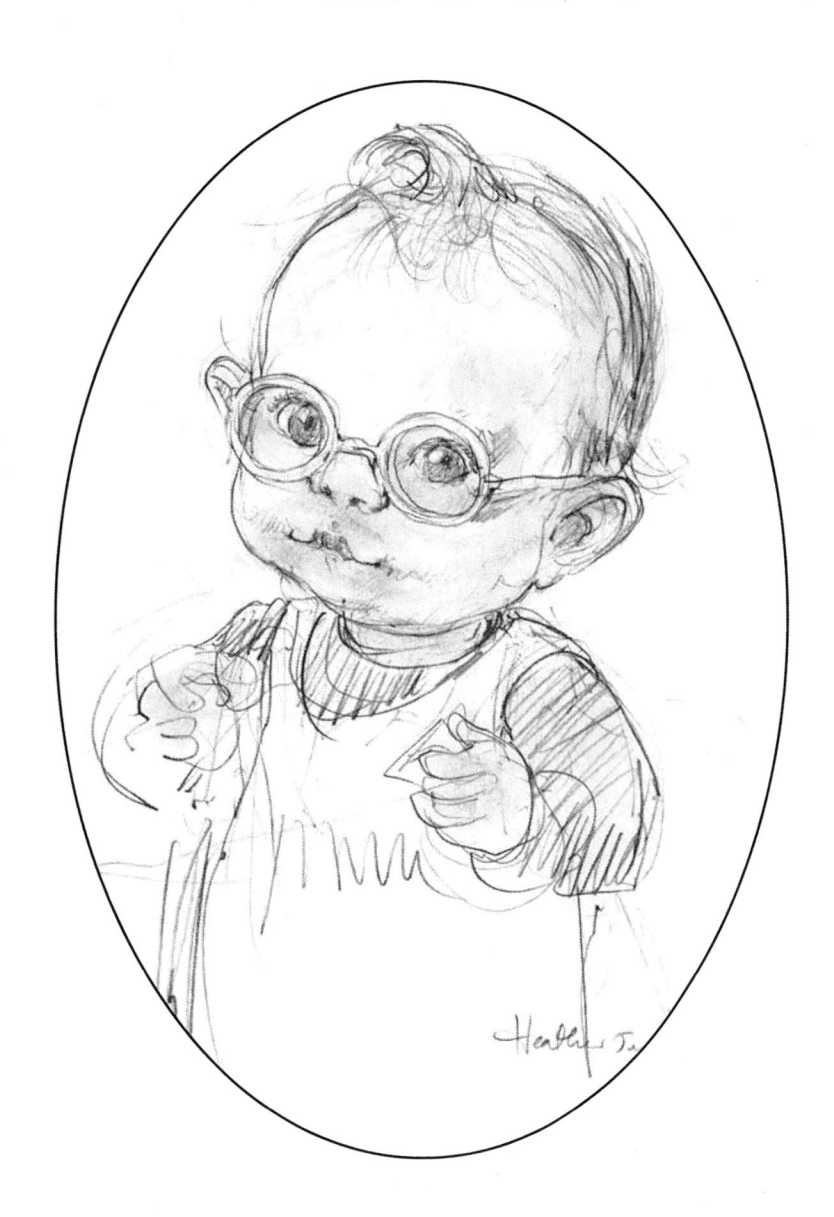

PART 2
VISION SCREENING BABIES
With Play

Table of Contents 95

How you can use Part 2 96

"Typical" Visual Development 97

Suggested Material List for Baby Vision Screening .99

Guidelines For Baby Vision Screening 100

Recording Form for Baby Vision Screening (PERMISSION TO REPRINT) 106

Feedback Form for Baby Vision Screening (PERMISSION TO REPRINT) 111

Spotting "Red Flags" Through Play Indicating Possible Vision Problems 115

Checklist: Spotting "Red Flags" (PERMISSION TO REPRINT) 117

Looking For "Red Flags" 120

What to Do About "Red Flags" 122

Bibliography 123

How you can use Part 2...

This is the playful part of this book. It was written for folks who don't have a vision background yet are responsible for screening vision of young children. It is designed to use as a screener to "red flag" possible vision problems. You don't need to get too involved with the details of the cause of a vision problem. However, you can look back into Part 1 for more information. Definitely find an experienced person to use as a resource.

You are presented with two sets of procedures that are easy and fun to use:
1. Baby Vision Screening
2. Spotting "Red Flags" through Play Indicating Possible Vision Problems

The checklist: Visual Development of "Typically" Developing Children", followed by a list of signs indicating children with possible visual deficits, are included to assist you in screening vision of young children. You need to know what "typical" visual development looks like so you can spot deviations. There are also some activities to assist in what to do with toys as you look for "red flags".

Permission is granted to reproduce the following forms in this Part 2:
1. Visual Development of "Typically" developing children
2. Recording Form Baby Vision Screening
3. Feedback Form for Baby Vision Screening
4. Checklist: Spotting "Red Flags"

If you want to ask questions don't hesitate in sending me a note at: Kathleen@visionkits.com

Hope this information is helpful....

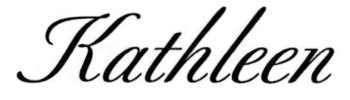

Kathleen

"TYPICAL" VISUAL DEVELOPMENT...

In order to assess vision you will need to review visual development of children who are developing typically so you can identify deviations from typical development. The following chart can be used as a guide. In some cases you may not be looking for deviations but for any signs of vision.

VISUAL DEVELOPMENT OF "TYPICALLY" DEVELOPING CHILDREN

AGE   **BEHAVIOR**

Birth - 1 month
- __Turns eyes & head to look at light sources
- __Appears to look through rather than at people
- __Black & white (high contrast) objects most interesting
- __PUPILS RESPOND TO LIGHT may be constricted 1st few weeks
- __FIXATION noted as child nurses with open eyes
- __MUSCLE BALANCE eye turn may be present, aligning later
- __HORIZONTAL PURSUITS with head movement, may be jerky
- __VERTICAL PURSUITS emerging
- __SHIFT OF GAZE from toy to toy slow with head movement
- __ACUITY poor due to immaturity of retina
- __CONTRAST SENSITIVITY poor due to immaturity of retina

2-3 months
- __Social smile by 3 months
- __Reaches toward & later grasps hanging objects.
- __FIXATION intense eye contact, interest in looking at moving lips
- __VERTICAL/HORIZONTAL PURSUITS with eyes only.
- __PERIPHERAL VISUAL RESPONSES within 60°
- __COLOR VISION prefers colored toys to black & white
- __ACCOMMODATES to different distances by 3 months
- __STEREOPSIS by 3 months

4 - 6 months
- __First time watching own hands is noted
- __Reaches toward faces & objects
- __Watches toys fall or roll away
- __VISUAL SPHERE gradually extends outward
- __SHIFT OF GAZE across midline
- __CONVERGENCE present by 6 months
- __PERIPHERAL VISUAL FIELDS responses within 180°
- __ACUITY recognizes distance objects, watches his or her hands.

7-10 months
- __Interest in pictures in books
- __Recognizes partially hidden objects
- __Pictures in books become interesting
- __FIXATION eye hand coordination improving
- __PERIPHERAL VISION symmetrical
- __ACUITY notices small objects like cereal & crumbs
- __PERCEPTION develops perception to form & size

11-12 months
- __Looks through window
- __Recognizes people, objects and pictures
- __Likes to play Peek-a-book
- __DEPTH PERCEPTION explores depth by looking into containers
- __COLOR PERCEPTION full color vision.

WHAT A ONE YEAR OLD WITH "TYPICAL" VISUAL DEVELOPMENT SHOULD BE ABLE TO DO...

- ✓ Accurately fixate without eye or head turn,
- ✓ Smoothly shift gaze across midline,
- ✓ Smoothly converge eyes to 3" from the nose.
- ✓ Smoothly follow moving toys horizontally & vertically with eye movement only.
- ✓ Visually accommodate, focus on objects at different distances.
- ✓ Upper visual fields reaching adult size and horizontal and lower fields smaller than adult size (Mohn & Hof-van-Duin, 1986)
- ✓ Acuity continues to improve as the retina matures.
- ✓ Contrast sensitivity reaching adult levels at about 3 years of age. (Hyvärinen, 1988).

- ✓ Lack of visual fixation of following by 3 months.
- ✓ Lack of accurate reaching for objects by 6 months.
- ✓ Persistent lack of eyes moving in concert or sustained "crossing" of 1 eye after 4-6 mos.
- ✓ Frequent horizontal or vertical jerky eye movements (nystagmus).
- ✓ Lack of a clear, black pupil (eg, haziness of the cornea, a whitish appearance inside the pupil, or a significant asymmetry of the usual "red eye" appearance of a flash photograph).
- ✓ Persistent tearing when the infant is not crying.
- ✓ Significant sensitivity to bright light (photophobia).
- ✓ Persistent redness of the normally white conjunctiva,
- ✓ Drooping of an eyelid sufficient to obscure the pupil,
- ✓ Any asymmetry of pupillary size or abnormalities to the eyes (Teplin, 1995).

BABY VISION SCREENING w/PLAY

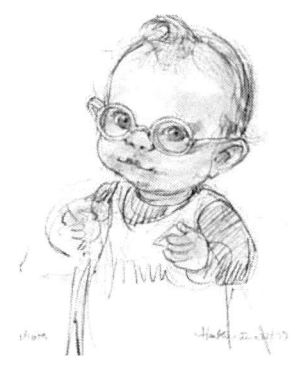

SUGGESTED MATERIAL LIST

APPEARANCE OF EYES & FIXATION
Black, White & Red Squeaky Puppet
Magnetic Wand
1" Metal Soccer Ball
2" Fixation Face Stick

FOLLOW MOVING TOY
2 Penlights
2 Animal Caps

SHIFT OF GAZE
Lighted Matching Toys

ACUITY
Soccer Balls: 1", 1½", 4"
0.5cm Candies
2 Pair One Eyed Glasses
LEA Grating Paddles
PÄIVI Book
LEA Symbol Single Symbol Book

PERIPHERAL RESPONSE TO TOYS
Creature on Clear Tube

PUPIL REACTIONS TO LIGHT
Penlight

Vision Associates   www.visionkits.com

BABY VISION SCREENING

RECORDING FORM GUIDELINES
Kathleen Appleby, M.A.

BEFORE YOU SCREEN

√ Take into consideration the child's age, handicaps and levels of functioning.

√ Note a baby's or multiple handicapped child's response patterns of breathing, quieting, smiling, babbling. This assists in detecting visual reactions to your toys.

√ Use child's own toy as a "looking motivator" if there is no interest in your toys.

√ Position the child so his/her body & head are supported.

√ Allow adequate response time. A multiple handicapped child may be slow to respond.

√ If baby is premature, use adjusted age to compare with the expected ranges.

APPEARANCE OF EYES & FIXATION

1. Observe what the child looks at and if he/she avoids looking.

2. Record the distance at which he/she stops looking at the toy.

3. If the child's eyes look as if they are in an unusual position, draw the eye positions on the form.

BE CONCERNED IF...

❑ The toy has to be closer than 3' before the child pays attention.

❑ The child avoids looking.

❑ A child fixates with head tilt or turn. Direct eye contact is absence as if the child is fixating beyond toy.

❑ An eye looks as if it turns in or out.

Vision Associates   www.visionkits.com

FOLLOW MOVING TOY

1. Use a motivating toy paired with sound or light if needed to attract a child's gaze.

2. Move the toy slowly horizontally & vertically while watching the child's eyes as he/she visually follows the toy, also observe the head position (pursuits).

3. Hold a toy, centered at eye level 18" from the child's nose and move it slowly toward the nose (convergence).

4. Note the distance the child's eyes stop turning in equally and smoothly as the toy gets closer and he/she stops fixating (convergence).

5. Hold the child's head still. if he/she moves it, and see if he/she can still follow the movement of the toy. See if the child's eyes can get into all extreme positions of gaze (full motility).

BE CONCERNED IF...

- ❑ After 1 year of age a child has to move his/her head, rather than use eye movement only. (Pursuits, #2 above)

- ❑ Child can not visually follow the toy in one or both directions. (Pursuits, #2)

- ❑ The eye movement is off pace with the movement of the toy. (Pursuits, #2)

- ❑ Eye movements are jerky or you note frequent breaks in fixation. (Pursuits, #2)

- ❑ he child stops fixating at the toy as it moves across midline by blinking or looking away. (Pursuits, #2)

- ❑ When the head is held the child struggles to move his/her body in order to watch the moving toy. (Pursuits, #2)

- ❑ The child's eyes stop turning in equally and smoothly or if he/she stops fixating at the toy when more than 3" from his/ her nose, if older than 6 mos. (Convergence, #3 & 4)

- ❑ Child can not get his/her eyes into all extreme positions of gaze. (Full Motility, #5)

SHIFT OF GAZE

1. Encourage the child to look straight ahead before you present the 2 toys. If using lighted toys you may have to dim the room lights.

2. Use two matching toys with sound and/or light and hold one in each hand, at child's eye level.

3. Place a toy in front of each eye on either side of midline equal distance apart.

4. Alternately light each toy to encourage the child to shift gaze from right to left and from left to right.

5. Reposition the toys above and below midline and alternately light each toy to see if the child can shift gaze from top to bottom and from bottom to top.

BE CONCERNED IF...

- ❑ The child can not smoothly shift gaze when looking from one toy to another. For example, the child's eyes may make several jerky movements before fixation on the second toy.

- ❑ The child can not shift gaze across midline without breaking fixation or blinking.

- ❑ he child needs to use head movement to shift gaze.

ACUITY

1. If possible try to cover an eye so you can evaluate each eye. Be sure the child stopped participating due to the task and not because he/she has lost interest.

2. <u>Functional Acuity:</u> Determine the smallest ball responded to and the furthest distance away from the child it was before he/she stopped looking.

3. On the recording form, put an "X" next to the size of the ball & write in the furthest distance the ball was from the child. Do both eyes & each eye individually. The child can wear the "one eyed sunglasses" to block an eye or use the Apple Cover or your finger.

4. Put an "X" next to the eye (or both eyes) that matches #3. If one eye had a different response write, next to the appropriate eye, the size and distance that eye demonstrated. For example: X BOTH   X RIGHT 4" ball at 3" LEFT.

5. <u>Grating Acuity:</u> To be used with babies up to 18 months of. When using the LEA Gratings, hold the gray paddle against a gray apron and put the largest grating behind it. Place them 22" from the child.

6. With equal movement pull each paddle out to either side of midline.

7. Observe the child's eyes to see if he/or she fixates at the grating paddle rather than at the gray paddle. Repeat moving the grating paddle to the other side.

8. Repeat using smaller and smaller gratings and note the narrowest gratings the child looked at before he/she stops fixating.

9. Write size of the grating (found on the paddle) next to the appropriate eye.

10. <u>Optotype Acuity:</u> See that the child can show you he can match the LEA symbols and identify them either by name or pointing to the matching one.

11. <u>Near acuity:</u> (Use with children who can identify pictures in a book by pointing.) Prepare the child for the **PÄIVI Book**, as per the directions in the book, and adapt them to his/her functioning levels. Have the child identify the symbols in the **PÄIVI Book**. Use the length of the opened book to measure 16" from the child if within the child's viewing distance. If not measure the distance the child prefers. 3 out of 5 symbols need to be identified to receive credit for each M-LEA Symbol size.

12. Write the M-size of the smallest LEA Symbol that the child could identify next to the appropriate eye on the Recording Form. Record the distance the book was held.

13. **Distance Acuity:** (Use with children 2 years and older, if appropriate.) Use the LEA Single Symbol book. Start with the 20/50 page. Use the "L" shaped cover to present the symbols one at time. Follow the directions included with the test.

14. Continue until the child can no longer get 3 out of 5 symbols correct.

15. Record the smallest LEA Symbol for each eye.

BE CONCERNED IF...

- ❑ The child does not look at the balls or needs to be closer than 3' away to see. (Functional acuity para #2, 3, & 4) above

- ❑ The child does not see the 1" ball at 10'. (Functional acuity #2, 3, 4)

- ❑ The child did not fixate on either the 4.0 or 8.0 cpcm LEA Grating Paddles at 22". (Grating acuity Paras #5-9)

- ❑ Child could not identify 3 out of 5 (1 M size symbols) at near. (Optotype acuity #11)

- ❑ Child could not identify 3 out of 5 (20/40 symbols) at 10'. (Optotype acuity #13 & 14)

- ❑ There is a difference between responses in each eye.

PERIPHERAL RESPONSE TO TOYS

1. Encourage the child to look straight ahead. Stand behind him/her and move a toy on a clear tube forward and around each side of the child, at eye level, and from above the head. Have someone face child to watch eye movement.

2. Note at what point in the field of vision the child turns to look at the toy. Mark an X on the drawing to identify that point.

BE CONCERNED IF...

- ❑ The child has a delay turning to look at the toy as it moves into range. He/she should turn soon after the first marking on the drawing. (6 mos. & up)

PUPIL REACTIONS TO LIGHT

1. Set the lights dim in the room and after a short while turn the lights on and observe the child's eyes. You should see the pupils get smaller and they should be equal in size.

2. **Direct:** . Do not do this area if child is seizure prone or on medication. Use a penlight and hold it about 18" from the child's nose and turn it on. If this is too intrusive turn the child toward the light of the window and watch the pupil responses. Both pupils should constrict equally, so each pupil should be the same size.

3. **Consensual:** Hold the edge of your hand between each eye to block the light. Quickly shine the penlight in the right eye and watch the response in the left eye. Repeat on the other side.

BE CONCERNED IF...

- ❑ The pupils do not get smaller in reaction to the light.

- ❑ Each pupil is a different size during the direct procedure. (#2)

- ❑ During consensual task eye that does not have a light in it doesn't get smaller. (#3)

BABY VISION SCREENING
RECORDING FORM
Kathleen Appleby, M.A.

CHILD'S NAME_____
BIRTHDATE_____ SCREENING DATE_____
SCREENING AGENCY_____
AGENCY ADDRESS_____
_____
AGENCY PHONE_____SCREEN-ER_____
PREMATURE?: ____YES ____NO, IF SO, ADJUSTED AGE:_____
MEDICATIONS?: ____YES ____NO, CHILD SEIZURE PRONE?: ____YES ____NO
HAS FAMILY BEEN TOLD CHILD HAS VISION PROBLEM?: ____YES ____NO ____NOT KNOWN
IF SO, DIAGNOSIS & TREATMENT:

APPEARANCE OF EYES & FIXATION

LOOKS AT: ____LIGHT ____FACES ____TOYS, AVOIDS LIGHT/GAZE: ____YES ____NO
DISTANCE STOPS LOOKING: _____ NEEDED TO RESPOND: ____MOVEMT, ____SOUND
VISUAL RESPONSE HAD TO BE PAIRED WITH: ____sound ____motion ____plain background
____good contrast ____color, Preferred: color_____ & object_____

POSITION OF EYES LOOK UNUSUAL
___NO ___YES ____NO RESPONSE

IF SO, DRAW EYE POSITIONS:
Child's Right   Child's Left

Eyes as you look at child
Some eye turn in early months expected

CONCERN: ___YES ___NO, DESCRIBE:

FOLLOW MOVING TOY

WATCH TOY MOVE FROM
SIDE TO SIDE (horizontal pursuits by 1 mo.):
 ____YES ____NO ____NO RESPONSE ____DIDN'T TRY ____NOT APPROPRIATE

WATCH TOY MOVE UP AND DOWN   (vertical pursuits by 3 mo.):
 ____YES ____NO ____NO RESPONSE ____DIDN'T TRY ____NOT APPROPRIATE

EYES ABLE TO GET INTO EXTREME POINTS OF GAZE:
 ____YES ____NO ____NO RESPONSE ____DIDN'T TRY ____NOT APPROPRIATE

WATCH TOY AS IT MOVES TO 3" FROM CHILD'S NOSE WITH SMOOTH & EQUAL INWARD EYE MOVEMENTS   (convergence by 6 mos.):
 ____YES ____NO ____NO RESPONSE ____DIDN'T TRY ____NOT APPROPRIATE

CONCERN: ____YES ____NO, DESCRIBE: **EMERGING:** ____YES ____NO, DESCRIBE:

SHIFT OF GAZE

LOOKS FROM ONE TOY/LIGHT TO ANOTHER (slow until 3 mos.):
 ____YES ____NO ____NO RESPONSE ____DIDN'T TRY ____NOT APPROPRIATE

SHIFTS GAZE ACROSS MIDLINE (by 3-6 mos.):
 ____YES ____NO ____NO RESPONSE ____DIDN'T TRY ____NOT APPROPRIATE

CONCERN: ____YES ____NO, DESCRIBE: **EMERGING:** ____YES ____NO, DESCRIBE:

ACUITY

SMALLEST BALL: ____.5cm ____ 1" ____ 1½" ____ 4"   FURTHEST DISTANCE_____
Check eye/s that apply to above & list any differences:
____BOTH ____RIGHT ____LEFT ____NO RESPONSE ____DIDN'T TRY ____N/A

AT 22" LAST GRATING FIXATED (4-16cpd by 18 mos):
____BOTH ____RIGHT ____LEFT ____NO RESPONSE ____DIDN'T TRY ____N/A

AT 16" SMALLEST SYMBOL NAMED (1M 20/50) (.63M 20/32)
____BOTH ____RIGHT ____LEFT ____NO RESPONSE ____DIDN'T TRY ____N/A

AT 10' child passed 20/40 line (3/5 right) __RIGHT __LEFT __BOTH (20/40 by 5 yrs)
____BOTH ____RIGHT ____LEFT ____NO RESPONSE ____DIDN'T TRY ____N/A

CONCERN: ___YES ___NO, DESCRIBE: EMERGING: ___YES ___NO, DESCRIBE:

PERIPHERAL RESPONSE TO TOYS

TURN TO TOY PRESENTED FROM EACH SIDE &
TOP & BOTTOM: (by 6 mos.)

Place an X at point child turns to toy:

Top View   Side View
PERIPHERAL VISION

CONCERN: ____YES ____NO, DESCRIBE:
(Include any central visual fields observations)

PUPIL REACTIONS TO LIGHT

PUPILS RESPOND EQUALLY IN SIZE TO LIGHTS TURNING ON OR OFF: ___YES ___NO
___NO RESPONSE ___DID'NT TRY ___SEIZURE PRONE

PUPIL RESPONSE: DIRECT: ___YES ___NO, CONSENSUAL: ___YES ___NO
CONCERN: ____YES ____NO, DESCRIBE:

SUMMARY & SUGGESTIONS

Check all areas of concern; these areas suggest possible vision problems.
* (Star) all areas of emerging skills.

___APPEARANCE/FIXATION   ___FOLLOWING MOVING TOY   ___SHIFT OF GAZE
___ACUITY: ___near ___distance ___PERIPHERAL RESPONSES ___PUPIL REACTION
REFER TO APPROPRIATE PROFESSIONAL: ___YES ___NO

SCREENER:_____
ADDRESS:_____
_____
_____
PHONE:_____
DATE:_____

Vision Associates   www.visionkits.com   K. Appleby, MA

BABY VISION SCREENING

FEEDBACK FORM
Kathleen Appleby, M.A.

CHILD'S NAME_____ BIRTHDATE_____
SCREENING DATE _____ SCREENING
AGENCY_____
ADDRESS_____
_____
PHONE_____
SCREENED BY_____
PREMATURE?: ____YES ____NO, IF SO, ADJUSTED AGE:_____
MEDICATIONS? ____YES ____NO ____NOT KNOWN
SEIZURE PRONE?: ____YES ____NO ____NOT KNOWN
HAS PARENT BEEN TOLD CHILD HAS VISION PROBLEM?: ____YES ____NO
IF SO, DIAGNOSIS & TREATMENT:
_____

The following is an explanation of <u>all</u> areas that are included in the Baby Vision Screening. The areas that have an **X** next to **CONCERN** indicate your child had difficulty with this area of the screening. It is to be noted that vision screenings measure performance and do not replace eye doctor examinations. Many non-visual factors may affect performance, such as motor abilities, processing skills, cooperation and cognitive abilities.

APPEARANCE OF EYES & FIXATION

__**CONCERN**   Observation of everyday activities gives insights into how children use their vision. We determine if a child looks at light, faces, toys, or avoids looking. The distance within which the child attends visually is also noted. When fixating it is noted if a child tilts or turns his/her head. Eyes should not appear to turn in or out.
COMMENTS:

FOLLOW MOVING TOY

__**CONCERN**   (Pursuits) We see if the child can visually follow a moving toy, with smooth eye movements, as it moves side to side, up and down, using eye movement without head movement.
__**CONCERN**   (Convergence) The child looks at an interesting toy as it moves closer to their nose. The child's eyes should turn in equally and smoothly as a toy move from 18" away to about 3" from the tip of his/her nose.
__**CONCERN**   (Limits of Gaze) When the child's head is held we observe to see if his/her eyes can get into all areas of extreme limits of gaze.
COMMENTS:

Vision Associates   www.visionkits.com   K. Appleby, MA

SHIFT OF GAZE

___CONCERN   the child should be able to smoothly shift gaze from one toy to another when the toys are placed to the right and left of midline and above and below midline.
COMMENTS:

ACUITY

___CONCERN   Acuity is the ability of the eyes to discern details and affects the overall ability to decipher what is seen. It is important to evaluate near and distance acuity and determine if responses are equal in each eye. Functional Acuity in young children can be measured using black and white balls of different sizes. Distance functional acuity can be observed by determining which size ball the child can see at 10' with each eye. Near functional acuity in each eye is determined when the examiner holds tiny candies at eye level for the child to see. Grating Acuity is noted when striped paddles of decreasing widths are presented in front of an infant simultaneously with a gray paddle (up to 18 mos). If the infant can see the stripes he/she is likely to look at them. Optotype Acuity tests are used to evaluate children who are able to match (by 18-24 mos.) They identify LEA Symbols at near and distance to determine the child's acuity.
COMMENTS:

PERIPHERAL RESPONSE TO TOYS

___CONCERN   Peripheral vision is noted by observing how far a toy (when presented from behind), coming from the sides and above and below, has to be moved toward the child's midline before it is noticed.
COMMENTS:

PUPIL REACTIONS TO LIGHT

___CONCERN   Normal pupillary responses include pupils getting smaller in bright light and bigger in dim light with equal sized pupils. Also eye responds when the light is only presented in the opposite eye.
COMMENTS:

SUMMARY & SUGGESTIONS

The checked areas indicate concern, based on the Baby Vision Screening.
* (Star) all areas of emerging skills.

  ____APPEARANCE/FIXATION   ____FOLLOWING MOVING TOY
  ____SHIFT OF GAZE   ____ACUITY: ____near ____distance
  ____PERIPHERAL RESPONSES   ____PUPIL REACTION

REFER TO APPROPRIATE PROFESSIONAL: ____YES ____NO
REFERRED TO:
COMMENTS & SUGGESTIONS:

SCREENER:_____
ADDRESS:_____
_____
PHONE:_____
DATE:_____

SPOTTING "RED FLAGS" THROUGH PLAY INDICATING POSSIBLE VISION PROBLEMS

This section was written for parents of early childhood children, for teachers who play and interact with children throughout the day, and for those folks responsible for screening children's vision. However, the information within is not to be used as a vision screening, as it is not inclusive of all areas of a screening. It is meant as a guide that offers additional observational information that might indicate a vision problem.

Vision is our primary learning channel so early identification of vision problems is extremely important. A good screening should include measuring acuity in each eye in order to spot possible amblyopia (Lazy Eye). Some vision problems go undetected even when children pass vision screenings. Undetected vision problems include observing how children's eyes work together, which can affect their visual motor skills, and school performance. As these children move up in the grades they may have difficulties keeping up in school when reading and writing demands increase in all subjects. Sherman, a researcher, found in a sample of 50 children with learning disabilities between the ages of 6 and 13 years old, that 96% had vision problems related to inefficiency of their eye movements.

It is also important to learn how a child with multihandicaps responds visually and how a child with limited vision uses his/her vision. How these children perceive their world can be impacted by their visual abilities. Early childhood teachers, therapists, and parents have great opportunities to observe children while interacting with them and watching them play. Hopefully you will learn to spot "red flags" for vision problems and learn ways to make adaptations to the environment to enhance the child's use of vision. If you see any "red flags" share the information with the children's parents/guardians so they can have discussions with their Pediatricians.

A baby developing in the "normal" progression will, by one year of age, be able to accurately fixate with aligned eyes, smoothly shift gaze across midline, converge his or her eyes to about 3" from the nose, and smoothly follow moving objects without head movement. Acuity continues to

improve as the retina (back of the eyeball) matures. Vision develops rapidly during the first year of life. Children with limited vision need visual stimulation to encourage visual development.

WHAT TO WATCH FOR IN PRESCHOOLERS

By following some simple steps you may be able to "red flag" children with undetected vision problems as they are engaged in activities. The first step is to become familiar with unusual behaviors that indicate possible problems. Take a look at children in action in order to spot these behaviors. Children with vision problems usually have to struggle harder in school than other children, even though they're smart. You know there's something not quite right, but you can't put your finger on what it is. They are often squirmy, can't sit still and require lots of attention; or they may be quiet and want to be left alone. They may get frustrated when cutting, coloring or playing with pegboards, and/or need to tilt or turn their heads during near activities.

In order to become familiar with unusual behaviors that indicate possible problems, use the Spotting "Red Flags" Indicating Possible Vision Problems Checklist to get a better idea if there are problems. Parents can complete the checklist at home and/or the school. Watch the child during everyday activities at home and/or in the classroom. Teachers and aides can use it in the classroom.

The checklist gives you a place to record any unusual behaviors you spot as children go about their daily activities. If the checklist is completed at school you may wish to share your observations with the child's parents. They may choose to talk with their pediatrician about any "checks". Check any of the following behaviors you see. Checked behaviors suggest the child may have a vision problem.

Spotting "Red Flags" Indicating Possible Vision Problems Checklist

by Kathleen Appleby, M.A.

CHILD'S NAME: _____ AGE _____ DATE: _____

RESPONDENT'S NAME: _____ PHONE: _____

A one year old child with "typically" developing vision can accurately fixate with aligned eyes, smoothly shift gaze, converge eyes, and smoothly follow moving objects with no head movement. Acuity and contrast sensitivity continues to improve as the retina matures

Please complete the above and check any area below that pertains.

APPEARANCE

_____ One eye turns in or out   _____ Closes an eye or tilts head for near tasks

_____ Red eyes, lids, or crust on eyelids   _____ Excessive blinking or tearing of eyes

NEAR & DISTANCE VISUAL ACUITY

_____ Holds things close to eyes   _____ Sits too close to the TV

_____ Thrusts head forward when looking at distance

LOW CONTRAST SENSITIVITY

_____ Needs more light to read than expected.

_____ Doesn't see soil spots on clothes or on counters

_____ Has trouble seeing outside on cloudy days

VISUAL FIELDS

_____ Difficulty with step downs   _____ Bumps into things

_____ Doesn't follow the words to the end of the sentence before going to the next.

ADAPTATION TO LIGHTING CHANGES

_____ Pauses when coming indoors on sunny days

_____ Slow adjustment to lighting changes, night travel difficulties

Vision Associates   www.visionkits.com

EYE TRACKING

_____Head moves instead of eyes when looking at pictures in books.

_____Loses place when moving his/her eyes along a line of small pictures.

_____Needs to use finger as a line marker.

_____Difficulty solving maze puzzles and games.

EYE TEAMING

_____Fatiques during near visual tasks, short attention span.

_____Difficulty judging where things are in space

_____Difficulty following flight of a ball.

Now you are ready to learn how to take a closer look at how young children fixate, move their eyes inward, shift their gaze, visually follow moving objects and identify smaller and smaller symbols at near in the PÄIVI Book. These skills can be observed in a play situation. The next step is learning How to Look For "Red Flags".

HOW TO LOOK FOR "RED FLAGS"

There are simple things you can do at home using everyday objects and toys. Select toys that are small, but not so small the children can't see them easily or that a child could swallow them. Use objects with interesting details so the child needs to look intently.

Suggested activities for each visual area are listed below and followed by what to expect from a child without vision problems. A list of behaviors that indicate a "red flag" comes next. Any "checked" behaviors indicate possible visual problems.

LOOKING FOR "RED FLAGS"

FIXATION When fixating at a small, interesting toy a child without vision problems has the ability to look directly at it without an eye turning in or out or turning his/her head.

(Hold a small toy at eye level and centered between the eyes, about 18" from the nose and observe the child's eyes and head position.)

BEHAVIOR INDICATES A "RED FLAG" IF:
____child does not look at the toy.
____child's eye is turned in or out.
____child tilts or turns head while looking at the toy.

VISUALLY FOLLOW A MOVING TOY

A child should be able to maintain fixation on a toy, without moving his head, as it moves in all directions in front of his face.

(Move a toy from right to left and left to right and then from up to down and down to up while watching the child's eyes, head & body.)

BEHAVIOR INDICATES A "RED FLAG" IF:
____child can't visually follow a toy without breaking fixation.
____child moves his or her head rather than using eye movement only, to watch toy.
____eye movements are jerky.

MOVEMENT OF BOTH EYES INWARD

A child should be able to keep looking at a toy with equal eye movement inward, as it is moved slowly toward his eyes until the toy is about 3" from his eyes.

(Hold a toy inline with the bridge of the child's nose about 18" away and move it slowly toward the child' eyes while watching his/her eyes.)

BEHAVIOR INDICATES A "RED FLAG" IF:
____child shows signs of eye fatigue, i.e., watery eyes, blinking or looking away.
____child's eyes stop turning in equally when the toy is further than 3" from nose.
____child moves his or her head to avoid looking.

SHIFT OF GAZE A young child is able to use smooth eye movements to shift fixation from one toy to another, without moving his head, when the toys are within his/her central visual viewing area.

(Hold two equally interesting toys, one in each hand, about 18" from the child's face and midway between each eye. Tell the child to look from one toy to another. You may need to alternately wiggle each toy telling the child to look at the toy that is moving.)

BEHAVIOR INDICATES A "RED FLAG" IF:

____ child can not smoothly shift gaze when looking from one toy to another.
____ child can not shift gaze across midline without moving his or her head.

ACUITY This is a near activity and does not look at distant viewing. A young child, when co-operating with the activity, should be able to located and identify all the **LEA Symbols** in the **PÄIVI Book** (at 16") as they get smaller, including those on page 11.

After Introducing the child to the LEA Symbols in the PÄIVI Book ask him/her to locate the bee and identify the Symbols as explained on each page. Continue through page 11. If the Symbols are too small turn to the low vision sized Symbols on page 12 so the child has success. Repeat page 11 while covering one eye at a time so you can compare the child's responses in each eye. Adjust presentation as per child's levels of functioning.

BEHAVIOR INDICATES A "RED FLAG" IF:

____ child can not locate the bee or the Symbols on any pages of the **PÄIVI Book.**
____ child needs to hold the book closer to 16" in order to see the Symbols.
____ child can identify Symbols on page 11 using one eye, but not with the other eye.
____ child has to turn or tilt head in order to see the Symbols.

WHAT TO DO ABOUT "RED FLAGS"

The information gained from these activities is only an observation of visual behaviors and is not a vision screening. The activities may assist in identifying children with poor visual skills. If red flags are noted, the parent/guardian may want to discuss them with the doctor. It is most important to determine why the child exhibited "red flags" and correct the problem, if possible. For example, if there were unequal responses in each eye using the PÄIVI Book and the doctor determines the child has amblyopia patching may be what the doctor requires. The following suggestions can be used to make things easier for the child while you wait to learn more about the cause of the "red flags" and if anything can be done to correct the problem.

ASSISTING CHILDREN WITH POOR VISUAL SKILLS

There is no "cookbook" to helping children since each child is unique. Pick and choose what works for your children.
- Allow extra time to complete near tasks, giving breaks every 5 minutes or so.
- Shorten the task when eye hand coordination is involved. For example, color only three shapes rather than five shapes, if the child struggles..
- Encourage using a finger as a guide when looking at rows of pictures in books.
- Use lots of materials to manipulate when learning new skills.
- Allow time to "check out" new things in a variety of ways: touch, sound, etc.
- Don't sit children facing windows since glare can affect visual performance.
- Another child can be a helping "buddy", when necessary. For example, when the child has to look up at the teacher's picture and then down at the book to find the matching picture, the buddy can help locate the matching picture.

You now have several ways to take a closer look at children's visual skills in the classroom and at home. Keep in mind the Academy of Ophthalmology and the American Optometric Association recommend that children should have eye examinations at about 6 months, 3 years, and 5 years of age. Since vision is the primary learning channel, taking a closer look is very important. So, don't be shy about taking a closer look at "red flags". Just think, a few minutes of fun can make a difference in a lifetime.

BIBLIOGRAPHY

Appleby, K. (1995) Play Vision assessment of functional vision. Manuscript for publication.

Appleby, K.(1997) Observing Visual Skills. Children and Families vol. XVI, No 2

Canadian Deaf-Blind and Rubella Associates, Ontario Canada, Vision screening in pre-school age children.

Cassin, B., Solomon, S., Rubin, M. (1990). Dictionary of Eye Terminology. Gainesville, Florida: Triad Publishing Co.

Sherman A. Relating vision disorders to learning disability. J Am Optom Assoc. 1973;44:140-45.

Scheiman M. (1997). <u>Understanding and Managing Vision Deficits A Guide for Occupational Therapists.</u> Thorofare, NJ: Slack, Inc.

Hyvärinen, L. & Appleby, K. (1995). Assessment prior to measurement of grating acuity in infants and children with handicaps. Manuscript for publication.

Hyvärinen, L., Assessment of visually impaired infants, (1994) Ophth Clinics of North American, Vol. 7:2.

Hyvärinen, L., Vision in children normal and abnormal. (1988) Canadian Deaf-Blind and Rubella Associates

Jan, J.E., Groenveld, A., Sykanda, A.M., Hoyt, C.S. (1987) "Behavioral Characteristics of Children with Permanent Cortical Visual Impairment." Developmental Medicine & Child Neurology, 25,755-762.

Jan, J., Groenveld, M., (1980) "Observations on the Habilitation of Children with Cortical Visual Impairment", Journal of Visual Impairment & Blindness, January 1990, 11-15.

Jan, J.E., Groenveld, M., (1993), Visual behaviors and adaptations associated with cortical and ocular impairment in children, Journal of Visual Impairment & Blindness, April, 1993, 101-105.

Jan, J., Whiting, S., Wong, P., Flodmark, O., Farrell, K., McCormick, A., (1985) "Permanent Cortical Visual Impairment In Children"/ Developmental Medicine & Child Neurology, 27, 730-739.

Steendam, M., (1989), Cortical Visual Impairment In Children, Royal Blind Society of N.S.W.

Teplin, S.W. (1995), Visual impairment in infants and young children, Infants and young children: An interdisciplinary journal of special care practices. 8, 18-45.